Personal Fitness Training

Beyond the Basics

Second Edition

Joe Cannon, MS

Copyright © 2019 by Joe Cannon

Joe Cannon's Website: Joe-Cannon.com

Published: Fauldhouse

Printed in the United States of America
Published December 2019

TABLE of CONTENTS

For Margaret Lynch Cannon, my 104-year-old
grandmother and oldest "client."
It was a pleasure.

Acknowledgments

No book is the work of only a single person but rather involves the collaboration of many others who worked behind the scenes, some without even knowing it. Let me take a moment to thank some of those people now.

As always, much thanks to Kelly Bixler, my proofreader and niece. It is good to have someone in the family to catch all of my typos.

This text would be much different if it were not for the efforts of Marcie Parke, the official illustrator of this book. Thanks for your hard work and dedication.

Thanks to my buddies, Chris Blessing, Paul Coppola, Tim DiFelice, Adam Freedman, and Bill Leinhauser for your friendship over the years and for helping me in your own unique ways.

Lastly, thanks to all of the fitness trainers who urged me to write this book. Your questions, emails, and comments over the years have been instrumental in helping me to write a more user-friendly book than I could have alone. Thank you all very much!

Start Reading Here

Congratulations! You are holding what I believe to be one of the most user-friendly books on personal fitness training in the world today. Within these pages, you will find the book that I have wanted to write for a very long time—a book that offers a "big picture" of personal training, addressing not only the scientific stuff that fitness trainers need to know but also the art of how to apply that science in the real world. I will endeavor to do this by aiming to converse with you as if I were sitting right next to you, sharing my own voyage of discovery, the facts I have learned over the years, personal stories, and even mistakes that I have made along the way.

Based on my own experiences, I have condensed some of the scientific concepts to reflect what I feel is most useful to fitness trainers. Where possible, I have also placed that science within the context of fitness and health to help foster learning and, hopefully, to spark your imagination.

Fitness professionals are primarily educators and often find themselves on the front lines fielding many questions. Because of this, I have purposely tried to answer some of those questions that I know you will one day be asked—and hopefully questions that you may have asked yourself from time to time.

Whether you are just starting out as a personal trainer or have been in the field for many years, it is my sincere hope that what I have created here will be of some help to you as you pursue your passion and help others achieve their dreams…

Joe Cannon

Let's Roll!

Chapter 1

BECOMING A PERSONAL TRAINER

There is a good chance that, if you are reading these words, you are either thinking about becoming a personal fitness trainer or you are already one and are looking for additional information. In either case, this chapter is beneficial to read because it will explain what it means to be a personal trainer and will offer information that may be helpful to both veterans and newcomers in the industry.

What Is a Personal Fitness Trainer?

Some may think the answer to this is a no-brainer, but I think it deserves mention. A personal trainer is a health and fitness professional who is usually contracted to perform private or semi-private exercise sessions with a person or small group of people. Notice the word "professional" in that definition. Personal trainers are professionals just like accountants, lawyers, business people, and others. Personal trainers are also members of the health care system along with physicians, nurses, physical therapists, pharmacists, chiropractors, massage therapists, and occupational therapists. While these professionals have skills and expertise that personal trainers may not have, it is also true that personal trainers have knowledge and proficiency in areas that these other professionals may not possess. Because of their connection to health, personal trainers should be familiar with how exercise impacts health. They should also be familiar with various principles of exercise science and how to apply those principles.

As professionals, personal trainers should strive to conduct themselves in a professional manner when they are in public or with clients. Several easy ways to do this include:

1. **Dressing appropriately.** If you are employed at a health club, adhere to its dress code. Maintaining proper attire helps members know who you are to prevent confusion. Baggy clothing is usually not appropriate, as it may become caught in equipment. Perfume and cologne should be used in moderation, if at all. Some people may be allergic to overly powerful cologne or perfume. In addition, if you are working with asthmatics, wear no scent, as it may exacerbate their condition. For those who are self-employed, dress modestly. The best and most functional outfits might include khakis, a collared shirt, and sneakers.

2. **Using business cards.** Business cards are one of the easiest ways to advertise yourself and your services as well as to tell the world that you have your act together.

3. **Being a people person.** You must enjoy helping people in order to be a fitness professional. You can have all the knowledge in the world, but if you cannot talk to others in a way that makes them feel comfortable, that will be problematic.

4. **Maintaining a professional relationship with clients.** Of course you are going to find some clients whom you will count among your friends—that is normal. Just be sure that, if you are working with a client as his or her personal trainer, you do not cross the line toward unprofessionalism. An example of such problematic behavior is intervening in marital

disagreements. It should go without saying, but I will say it anyway—personal trainers must not have inappropriate relations (that means sex!) with clients! As a personal trainer, you represent an entire industry of thousands of people, and what you do reflects upon everyone else in the industry. Aside from embarrassing all parties, serious violations of professional conduct can also result in the revocation of your fitness certification. If you are serious about being a fitness professional and are passionate about your trade, then there is a good chance that you may go from relative obscurity to being well known. You do not want anybody to be able to drag skeletons out of your closet that hold you back on the path toward success.

5. **Maintaining a network with other health professionals.** No personal trainer knows everything or can be all things to all people. To give people the best possible service, all personal trainers should have contacts with other health care professionals when their client's needs fall outside the scope of a personal trainer's practice. Registered dietitians, physical therapists, occupational therapists, massage therapists, and chiropractors are all good examples.

6. **Keeping personal information private.** Because personal training is *personal*, you will likely be privy to an assortment of personal information regarding your clients. While they may share some information in confidence, you may simply overhear other things in passing. It is important that all of this information remains in your "lockbox." Divulging personal information is the fastest way to lose a client and to gain a bad reputation.

7. **Staying educated.** People are pretty smart, so as a fitness professional, you will be asked all sorts of questions. Obviously you cannot know everything, but the best way to be prepared is to keep up with what is going on in your field. Reading books, attending seminars, and subscribing to trade journals are some of the easiest ways to stay on top of things.

PT or CPT?

Some personal trainers refer to themselves as "PTs." This makes sense since the two first letters in personal training are "P–T." That being said, the abbreviation "PT" is usually understood by the public to mean "physical therapy." To avoid confusion, the acronym "CPT," which stands for "certified personal trainer," was devised. Some personal trainers even have the letters "CPT" behind their names and on their business cards. When in doubt, it is probably wise not to list what you do as "PT," as doing so may cause confusion or even annoy physical therapists, who used the acronym first.

Where Do Personal Trainers Work and How Much Do They Make?

According to the US Bureau of Labor and Statistics, there are over 250,000 certified fitness trainers in America.[40] The actual number of personal trainers may be much higher than this given that some may not be certified. Personal trainers are employed in a number of fields, with the majority being employed in fitness centers and health clubs. Salaries for personal trainers can vary with location as well as with education and experience, but according to the US Bureau of Labor and Statistics, the average annual income for trainers in 2012 was about $31,000.[40] While that may not seem like much, the top 10% of personal trainers in America earned over $66,000.[40] For trainers who are self-employed, the amount can be even higher.

What Is Better: A Degree or Certification?

For those just starting (and for those who have been in the field for a while), the question often arises as to whether a college degree or fitness certification is better for practicing personal training. Some personal trainers do, indeed, have college degrees, and this may appeal to some employers and to clients. However, a college degree does not necessarily mean that you deeply know personal training. It is a fact that many college exercise degree programs either do not teach or spend very little time teaching the "art" of personal training. For this reason, many employers recommend that their personal trainers have fitness certifications as well.

Today there are hundreds of fitness certifications from which to choose. Some of the larger and more widely recognized organizations include the American Aerobics Association International/International Sports Medication Association (AAAI/ISMA), American College of Sports Medicine (ACSM), American Council on Exercise (ACE), Interactive Fitness Trainers of America (IFTA), International Sports Sciences Association (ISSA), National Academy of Sports Medicine (NASM), and National Strength and Conditioning Association (NSCA). For more info on fitness organizations, see my reviews at Joe-Cannon.com.

While all certifying organizations essentially teach similar topics, they may differ in the amount of attention that they devote to various subjects and in the weight that they give to different topics on their certification exams. Some involve self-study, while others are classroom-based, and others may require a college degree before you are allowed to take the exam. Many require a current CPR/AED certification as well. Certifications also differ in cost. It is a myth that expensive certifications are better than less costly certifications. At the end of the day, knowledge assimilated is more important than one's certification organization of choice.

Obtaining a CPR/AED Certification

In addition to a fitness certification, it is wise to also have a CPR certification. Obtaining this certification before signing up for a fitness certification is a good idea, as many organizations require this as a prerequisite for taking their test. Also, many health clubs require a current CPR certification prior to employment. CPR certifications are relatively inexpensive, costing around $50 in some areas. Both the American Red Cross (www.redcross.org) and American Heart Association (www.americanheart.org) websites let people connect with certifications in various regions. CPR classes are also offered at local colleges, hospitals, YMCAs, and fire stations.

Often, the CPR certification is combined with an AED certification. AED stands for "automated external defibrillator." This is a portable device which, in the event of a heart attack, can help keep a person alive until help arrives. Many health clubs have AEDs on site and require staff and managers to be properly trained to use them. To obtain such training, contact either the Red Cross or the American Heart Association through the websites listed above.

What Is the Best Certification?

People often wonder which is the best fitness certification. Honestly, the lay public usually does not know one certification from another. Moreover, some certifications, while very good, assume that the student has advanced knowledge prior to taking a certification exam or discusses topics using language that only a genius such as Albert Einstein could understand. I personally have textbooks that I have had to read a few times before comprehending what the author is talking about! The bottom line is that one should not get hung up on which is the best certification. The trick is to find a certification that is reputable, teaches the concepts necessary for working safely with others, allows for relatively easy re-certification, and (in my opinion) is cost effective for your budget.

Whichever certification you obtain, the most important thing that you can do is to continue educating yourself. A certification by itself only demonstrates that you have met the minimum requirements to become a personal trainer—it does not mean that you know everything. You would not want a doctor who only met minimum requirements, would you? Of course you would not! The same goes for your clients. Having a certification plus six-pack abs may get you a few clients, but if you cannot accurately answer a question such as "Why does my urine look like Coca Cola after I work out," you are at a big disadvantage and probably will not retain those clients for long. Knowledge is power, and is more valuable to people than the size of one's biceps. Consumers are very smart these days, and they look for professionals who can save them time while working out, but also as they search for answers regarding health. For more on this topic, see my post "What's the Best Personal Training Certification?" which is found at my website, Joe-Cannon.com. Also, keep reading for the answer to the coke-a-cola urine question…

Chapter 2

WHAT TO DO WHEN YOU GET A NEW CLIENT

For those just starting out in the business of personal training, one of the most frequently asked questions is, "What do I do when I get a new client?" This makes perfect sense, especially because many certifications and college degree programs tend to focus only on the "nuts-and-bolts" science behind personal training. While personal training is very science-based, the art of applying these principles and executing training sessions should not take a back seat. Both are closely intertwined. All the knowledge in the world will not help if you cannot gain a client and foster a working relationship. To address this issue, we will now review some of the steps that a trainer should take when he or she gets a client—whether it is the very first personal training client or the one hundredth.

The Initial Interview

The initial interview is the first meeting that you will have with a new client. This time can be used to gather valuable information as well as to demonstrate professionalism to the new client. Unless the client specifically asks you to call them by his or her first name, using formal modes of address is always preferable. Whenever possible, the initial interview should be conducted in a private area such as an office. This is because the client will be divulging sensitive private information. In addition, conducting the interview in private can also help reduce any uneasiness that the client may feel during any fitness testing that occurs. Taking circumference or body fat measurements in a public area is one of the fastest ways to make a new client feel uneasy. While this may not be an issue for trainers who go to people's homes, in gyms and health clubs with limited space, this can be a difficult obstacle to overcome.

Another advantage of the initial interview is that it provides a time for the trainer and client to get to know each other by engaging in conversation. On the surface, this may seem secondary to the main goals of the interview, but this can help the trainer gather valuable information. It is sometimes said that over 80% of a spoken sentence is nonverbal (i.e., is influenced by body language). Nonverbal cues such as poor posture, a lack of eye contact, and folding of the arms may indicate a client's struggle to feel confident. For example, someone who timidly sits in a chair without removing his or her coat indoors may be depressed or nervous. The ability to recognize these sorts of nonverbal signs is an invaluable tool to which many pay little attention.

During the initial interview (if not before), fitness professionals should provide the client with their personal contact information such as a cell phone number and an email address. Providing this information can help the client to schedule sessions or to cancel them if an emergency arises. Ideally, only the number of the phone that the trainer is most likely to answer should be given. Providing several phone numbers increases the chances of a missed call, which may cause trainer or client to miss an appointment. Also, the phone number given should have voicemail so that clients can leave a message if needed. Your personal voicemail greeting should be professional and easy to understand. Likewise, it is in the trainer's best interest to provide a professional, easy-to-spell email address such as "YourName@gmail.com." Email addresses that are lewd or suggestive are inappropriate for business purposes and are one of the fastest ways to make a bad impression on a new client.

The Health History Form

A man joins a health club and hires a personal trainer to help him get back in shape. About 10 minutes into their first workout, the man starts to look tired and has to sit down. The trainer becomes concerned and asks whether the man is ok, to which the man replies, "I'll be ok in a few minutes—I had open heart surgery three weeks ago and I'm still recovering!" Now, you can imagine the shock on the face of the personal trainer who, until that very moment, had no idea that the man had undergone such a major surgical procedure! This is actually a true story that was told to me by the personal trainer himself! I mention this because it highlights one of my rules of personal training: Never work with someone until you know his or her personal health history.

The fact cannot be stated enough that personal trainers MUST know the clients with whom they are working. Do not assume that people are healthy simply because they are in a health club or "look" fit. A topic that is not often talked about is that numerous at-risk individuals walk the floors of every health club in the world. People have died in health clubs, too. I say this not to frighten you, but to arm you with the knowledge that this is true so that you may be better prepared if (and when) you encounter one of these individuals. How can you identify high-risk people? Have them complete a health history questionnaire. All health history forms will probably have the same major sections, including personal contact information, personal and family health history, medication usage, and fitness history.

Personal Contact Information

This section of a health history form includes data such as name, address, phone number, email address, the name and phone number of the primary care physician, and emergency contact information. It is very important that all personal and medical history data be kept private. Fitness professionals should refrain from discussing a client's personal or private information with other colleagues in a way that would allow for the client to be identified. In addition, the client's specific health conditions and other personal data should not be discussed in public settings. Personal trainers should keep all of their clients' information in an organized and secure filing system such as a lockable filing cabinet. This is especially important for hospital-based fitness centers that may be subject to special privacy regulations.

Personal Health History

This section is where you collect information on the client's current and past health status. It is here that questions pertaining to medical conditions and injuries are asked. Other questions can include those pertaining to cholesterol levels, blood pressure, and cigarette smoking habits.

Fitness professionals who encounter clients with serious medical issues such as heart disease, diabetes, and other conditions should refer them to a primary care physician to obtain a written approval note before exercise training begins. This serves not only as an extra measure of safety for the individual, but also may help the fitness professional in the event of future litigation. Obtaining a note from a qualified medical professional can also been viewed as a marketing opportunity for personal trainers. As many know, it can be difficult to schedule a meeting with a physician because they are busy with patients, paperwork, and other demanding, time-consuming tasks. By referring high-risk people back to their physicians prior to training, you open up an opportunity for various physicians to get to know you better. More importantly, you demonstrate to local physicians your level of competency and the care that you provide for their patients.

Family Health History

Several years ago, I was told by the management of the health club where I worked that they would no longer need me to work on the weekends because the club was not very busy during those times. I felt that it was a mistake not to have any fitness staff on duty, but for reasons only management can answer, the club stuck to its guns. Unfortunately, about a month later everyone's worst nightmare came true when a man in his mid-30s died while working out at that very club over the weekend. While you might think that is the end of the story, it is not. I later learned that the man had a brother who, just a few years before, also died from a heart attack. I share this sad story to emphasize the importance of knowing the health history of a client's immediate family members. In general, those whose mother, aunt, or sister died suddenly or had a heart attack before the age of 65 or whose father, uncle, or brother passed away or had a heart attack before the age of 55 may be at an increased risk of early death from heart disease.[1] These people should be referred to a physician prior to training. In addition, knowledge of family health issues may enable the trainer to help his or her client more fully. For example, if a family history of osteoporosis is known, it may be possible to use exercise to reduce the chance of its development in the client in the future.

Heart Disease Risk Factors[1]

Risk Factor	Specific Information
Family History	Heart attack, heart disease surgery, or sudden death before the age of 55 in father or immediate relative (son, brother) or before the age of 65 in mother or other immediate relative (sister, daughter)
Cigarette Smoking	Someone who is a current smoker or who quit smoking in the past 6 months
High Blood Pressure	Blood pressure greater than 140/90 mm Hg or someone on medications for high blood pressure
High Cholesterol Levels	Total cholesterol greater than 200 mg/dl or HDL less than 40 mg/dl or someone taking medications for high cholesterol. Also someone whose LDL cholesterol is greater than 100 mg/dl
Obesity	Having a BMI greater than 30 kg/m^2 or having a waist circumference greater than 100 cm
Non-Active Lifestyle	Those not regularly engaging at least 30 minutes of sustained activity most days of the week

Note: An HDL of 60 mg/dl or better is considered a "negative risk factor" for heart disease. In other words, this lowers the chance that heart disease may develop.[1] Aerobic exercise does a good job of raising HDL.

Who Is Low-Risk and Who Is High-Risk?

By using the preceding table of heart disease risk factors, it is possible to estimate a person's risk for heart disease.[1] The following table can help us develop a better idea of who is low- and high-risk according to the risk factors just described.

Low Risk	Children, adolescents, men younger than 45, and women younger than 55 who have no symptoms of heart disease and have no more than 1 risk factor
Moderate Risk	Men 45 or older, women 55 or older, or those who have 2 or more risk factors
High Risk	Persons who have heart disease, diabetes, or lung disease or those who have one or more heart disease signs or symptoms

Medication Use

Fitness professionals are generally not physicians or pharmacists and are not expected to understand how medications work. That being said, it is a good idea to inquire about the types of medications that people are taking because it can help you better address their needs. For example, some medications (e.g., beta blockers) can make it harder for people to exercise. This is important information to know when designing an exercise program. When discussing medications, the conversation should be viewed as another opportunity to identify high-risk people. When you encounter people who are taking medications to treat serious conditions like high blood pressure, diabetes, heart disease, kidney disorders, or cancer, they should be referred back to a physician and instructed to obtain a written note from the doctor offering medical clearance to exercise. The approval note should be kept in the person's file. Personal trainers, like all fitness professionals, are members of the health care continuum, a spectrum of diverse medical and healthcare practitioners that works best when the client's primary care physician is kept informed about what his or her patient is doing. Exercise can generally help improve overall health, but some people should obtain medical clearance before they begin an exercise program.

Conditions That Require a Physician's Approval*

Heart disease	Chest pain at rest	Emphysema
High blood pressure	Chest pain during exercise	Pregnancy
Kidney disorders	Diabetes	Cancer
Prior heart attack	HIV/AIDS	Asthma
Pacemaker	Morbid Obesity	Sedentary lifestyle
Heart surgery	Early death of parents	Stroke

* This is a partial list

Some health history forms may also inquire about the use of dietary supplements. Studies show that most Americans take supplements ranging from multivitamins to exotic herbs, minerals, and other products reputed to help any number of conditions. Some health clubs also sell supplements. For the record, there are good supplements and less ideal varieties. The trick is to figure out which are better options for health. Many trainers may be ill-equipped to deal with this issue, which is why I recommend exercising caution, especially because supplements can interact with medical issues and medications. Something that is presumably "all natural" is not necessarily safe for everybody. For more on this topic, see my post "Should Personal Trainers Recommend Supplements?," which may be found at Joe-Cannon.com.

Fitness History

Obviously, it is a good idea to know about the past (and present) experiences that your client has had with exercise. Questions for this section can include:

> ➢ What types of physical activity do you enjoy?
> ➢ What physical activities have you done in the past?
> ➢ Do you participate in any sports?
> ➢ Do you have difficulty performing any physical activity?

Questions like these help tease out information about a person's likes and dislikes and can assist with designing an effective exercise program that is not only enjoyable, but that also addresses the person's specific needs. For example, for people indicating that they play a particular sport or activity, the trainer may incorporate movements that can strengthen muscles to help them play their sport better while also reducing the risk of injury.

The PAR-Q

Besides the health history form, one may also wish to administer a separate document called the "PAR-Q." PAR-Q stands for "Physical Activity Readiness Questionnaire." Basically, the PAR-Q is a one-page form that can help identify people who may not be suitable for exercise. The PAR-Q is appropriate for people 15–69 years of age and provides the very minimum amount of information that should be obtained prior to working with someone.[1] The PAR-Q, however, is not foolproof and should be just one component of a comprehensive screening process that also includes a health history form. The PAR-Q consists of a short series of easy-to-understand questions. The bottom line is that if the person answers "yes" to any of the questions, then there is a possibility that he or she may have significant medical issues and should see a doctor before starting an exercise program.

PAR-Q Questions[1]

1. Has your doctor ever said that you have a heart condition and that you should only do physical activity recommended by a doctor?
2. Do you feel pain in your chest when you do physical activity?
3. In the past month, have you had chest pain when you were not doing physical activity?
4. Do you lose your balance because of dizziness or do you ever lose consciousness?
5. Do you have a bone or joint problem that could be made worse by a change in your physical activity?
6. Is your doctor currently prescribing drugs (for example, water pills) for your blood pressure or heart condition?
7. Do you know of any other reason why you should not do physical activity?

The actual PAR-Q form can be viewed online. Simply entering the phrase "PAR-Q and You" into any major search engine will bring up the form. Aside from its use by fitness professionals, health clubs should also use this document. If all new health club members completed the PAR-Q prior to joining a health club, it might help decrease the number of high-risk people who joined without a doctor's approval.

Additional Forms

The Waiver

Before the first training session occurs, all clients should complete a legally binding waiver of liability, sometimes called a Release form. This form can help protect the fitness professional if something unfortunate occurs during training. Having a properly worded waiver can help reduce the likelihood of lawsuit. Most fitness centers have carefully worded waivers that all members sign prior to joining, and some fitness centers may even have additional personal trainer waivers that people sign prior to working with a personal trainer. If you are working in a health club, ask the manager or owner about their specific guidelines regarding waivers. Self-employed personal trainers must have their own waiver. Regardless of whether you are self-employed or work at a health club, waivers, like all client information, should be kept in a safe, secure place.

Ideally, waivers should be drawn up by an attorney in your state who has knowledge of Contract Law and the health and fitness industry. When searching for a lawyer, you may want to ask prospective attorneys whether they have previously created documents such as waivers for fitness professionals.

The size of the words on some waivers that I have seen is so small that people may have difficulty reading them. Thus, the font size should be legible. You may want to have both hard copies as well as a PDF file stored on your computer. This will enable you to email the waiver to clients if necessary. Your attorney can help you with this.

It is also important that the fitness professional explain the nature of the waiver to the client so that he or she understands what the document means. When discussing the waiver, do not downplay its significance. In other words do not say, "This is something that I have to do; it really doesn't mean much." By signing the waiver, the client is essentially waiving many (but not all) of his or her rights to take legal action. This is very significant! Downplaying the significance of the waiver might open up a legal loophole that could lead to negative outcomes for the trainer in the event that he or she is ever taken to court. An attorney can offer advice on the best way to explain the waiver to people. Also, keep in mind that waivers may not protect a fitness trainer in all circumstances, specifically if the professional is performing tasks that fall outside of his or her scope of training practice (e.g., recommending dietary supplements).

Lastly, keep in mind that laws vary from state to state. A waiver created for a fitness center or personal trainer in Texas may not be sufficient in Massachusetts. Thus, it is not a good idea for trainers to copy a previously used waiver found on the Internet. Hiring an attorney is truly the best course of action. Fitness trainers are usually not lawyers and are not expected to be, and an attorney can help save a lot of time and legal fees down the road.

Liability Insurance

Just as you probably have insurance for your car and health, personal trainers should also have liability insurance. While personal trainers who work at health clubs may be covered by the club's policy (check to make sure), self-employed personal trainers MUST have their own liability insurance.

While not the norm, some health clubs may allow outside trainers (who are not employees) to work with clients at their facility. In this instance, the club will require the trainer to provide not only a copy of his or her fitness and CPR certifications, but proof of liability insurance as well. Many companies exist that can provide liability insurance, and the organization by which a trainer is certified can often provide guidance in choosing in the right plan. Prices usually range from $200–$500 per year. Keep in mind that liability insurance may not cover all possible incidents.

Trainer/Client Agreement

The agreement between the client and the trainer is a document that is sometimes used to help outline the responsibilities of both parties. It may not be legally binding; however, the client and trainer both normally sign the form to ensure that the client follows through on his or her commitment. This form contains information regarding dressing properly for workouts, showing up on time, giving a reasonable amount of notice (that you specify) if he or she (or the trainer) must cancel a workout, and so on.

Goal Sheet

Obviously, the fitness professional should know the reasons why the client has sought out his or her services, and this is where a goal sheet comes in handy. Unfortunately, it has been my personal observation that many trainers miss the power of learning about goals. This is probably because, as many fitness professionals will tell you, most people have the same goals—tone up, lose weight, or build muscle. After seeing the same goals day after day or month after month, trainers may begin to take them for granted. That being said, I would like to suggest a new way to gather information on goals. Have all clients write a paragraph for each goal that they have. Have them list all of the reasons why they want to attain their goals and advise them to be as specific and honest as possible. You might assign this as homework since it will take them some time to complete. Reassure them that nobody will ever view what they have written and that their information will be kept confidential. This is crucial because they will probably write their private, innermost thoughts and feelings. Having people commit to writing their goals in this way helps them take ownership of those goals and enables them to take a small step toward pursuing their fitness aims. Over time, this makes them more likely to take the bigger step of achieving their goals. If they list more than one goal, ask them to prioritize them. For example, put a "1" next to the goal that is most important.

When you have a client's written goals, review them on a regular basis (e.g., once a week). This should be done in private. Ask the individual to identify feelings of triumph during the previous week (this helps reinforce good behavior) and to discuss any setbacks. Write everything down and store the information in the client's file, which should be kept in a locked area such as a file cabinet.

When dealing with setbacks, try to design strategies to avoid or better deal with problem areas in the future.

Nutrition Assessment

Some fitness professionals also include a sheet on which clients can list the types of foods that they eat. This is sometimes called a 3-day or week-long food journal. Various nutrition websites and apps can also help track this data. Some fitness centers use nutrition tracking as an opportunity to introduce members to other services that they offer, such as nutritional counseling or special educational programs geared toward weight loss. Whatever the reason, if a trainer encourages clients to do this, he or she must make sure that they only list foods eaten during "typical" days. Foods eaten on special events such as weddings should not be listed. For more information on nutrition and sports nutrition, read my book entitled *Nutrition Essentials*, available at www.Joe-Cannon.com.

Summary: Getting Off to a Good Start with New Clients

1. Arrive early for appointments
2. Listen to clients needs and concerns
3. Have all relevant forms handy and ready for the client
4. Provide personal contact information
5. Be professional

After the First Meeting: What Is Next?

Now that you have met with your client and he or she has completed all of the necessary paperwork, what should happen next? Let us assume that you both have agreed to meet three times a week. After you agree to meet at a specified time, arrive for the session at least 10 minutes early if you work in a health club. That way, you have a little time to get everything that you need before the session begins. If you are a fitness trainer who goes to people's homes or offices, arrive on time for the session, if not a few minutes early. If you are going to such private spaces, odds are that the client will be working on other things before you arrive, so if you arrive too soon, it may complicate his or her schedule. Usually, arriving five minutes prior to the session is acceptable. If you are going to be late for a session, call the client and inform them or, if you work at a health club, call the front desk and have them notify the client when he or she arrives. Adding the club's number in your cell phone makes this easy and efficient. When you meet the client, shake his or her hand and address the person in a formal manner (using "Mr." or "Mrs.," for example).

You should be appropriately dressed for the session. In other words, wear the club's uniform or, if you are a self-employed trainer, wear something casual yet professional such as a warm-up suit or khakis and a shirt. Breath mints or gum may also be something to consider (after all, personal training is personal!). Clothes that emulate the latest urban fashion trends are usually not appropriate. Think about it: if you are training a 50-year-old businessman, will he be able to identify with a trainer who looks like he or she just walked out of a music video? Probably not! In fact, that guy probably would not hire that trainer. In personal training, appearances do matter to a certain degree. While looks are not the primary factor, when it comes to first impressions, people unfortunately do tend to judge a person by the clothing that he or she wears.

Let us assume that you have already developed the exercise program for your client and are taking him or her through it. Before the workout begins it is always a good idea to ask the person how he or she is feeling. I usually make it a point to ask people whether they have any pains, especially in the neck, shoulders, elbows, low back, knees, or ankles. By asking them this, I hope to remind them of any other issues, injuries, or problems that they should communicate to me before the workout begins. I do this for all clients, whether I see them infrequently or several times a week.

All workouts should have a warm-up period of 5–10 minutes to help prepare the body for exercise. You can be present during the warm-up or advise the client to perform it him or herself. For people with special needs, it is a good idea to be present for the warm-up to ensure that they remain safe. You will need your workout sheet to record the weights, repetitions, sets, and other notes as the client performs the designated exercises. Record all of your client's workouts. If you have several clients, this makes it easier for you to remember who did what. Hollow clipboards in which you may store workout sheets, pens, and other supplies can be purchased at office supply stores. Tablet computers may also be used to serve this purpose. The information that you track for clients can be a valuable motivational tool. Not only are workout sheets pretty easy to make on the computer, you can also download templates from the Internet.

If you are working in a health club, you are going to have to share the road not only with other trainers but also with other club members. Most people in health clubs are pretty courteous to each other and do not mind sharing equipment. If you encounter a member resting on a piece of equipment that you want to use, simply ask the member if you can "work in." Most times people will comply. If you use equipment like dumbbells or medicine balls, return them to their proper place before moving to another exercise. Leaving unattended fitness equipment out in the open is a safety hazard.

To Touch or Not To Touch?

Personal training is *personal,* and there may be times when it is necessary to touch the client in order to spot him or her or to provide guidance regarding proper alignment and form. It is important to remember that some people may not feel comfortable with being touched by another person, especially by someone whom they hardly know. Touching someone who feels that the touching was inappropriate could lead to disciplinary action or worse yet—legal action! I personally have encountered fitness trainers who do not touch *any* of their clients because of the stigma attached to it. Having said this, it is a good idea to explain the nature of spotting and occasional touching during the initial interview to familiarize the client with the process. During sessions, when you feel that touching is necessary, ask first whether it is ok. In reality, there is no perfect way to address this situation. I believe that by conducting oneself in a professional manner and by forming true friendships with clients, a trainer may avoid many problems that may arise as a result of spotting clients.

When you are working with a client, make sure that he or she can exit an exercise machine safely. When I worked in health clubs, I occasionally saw trainers who seemed determined to quickly move to the next exercise before the client was ready. They did this probably because they wanted to provide the best service to their clients and prepare the next exercise station before the client arrived. This is well intentioned, but keep in mind that clients may not be as familiar with fitness equipment as trainers. Some fitness machines are pretty complicated and people may have difficulty with dismounting a piece of equipment. This can be particularly true for people with special needs, seniors, those with fibromyalgia, or those who are overweight.

It is important to remember that clients should have your undivided attention during sessions. This means that you should never text or take cell phone calls while working with clients. Doing so may lead to reprimands by gym management. That said, this can sometimes be a challenge, especially if you work in a busy health club where other members may approach you to ask for your advice. Some clubs may try to deal with the situation by having the staff wear different colored shirts to alert members to who is considered "fitness floor staff" and who is working as a personal trainer. Regardless, if you are working with someone and are approached by another member, be courteous and tell them that you can help them when you are finished with your client. If the need is immediate, refer them to a fitness staff member who is on duty.

When you have completed your session with the client, set a date for your next meeting if you have not already done so, and record the date in your day planner. If you are seeing clients back-to-back, give yourself a few minutes between appointments. That will give you time to prepare for the next person. Because it is likely that you will be touching various pieces of equipment during the day, it is a good idea to wash your hands between clients, as fitness equipment may harbor germs.[20] If washing is not possible, carry an alcohol-based product with you. While this may seem like overkill to some, no one wants to accidently transmit infections to clients! Also, as all trainers know, if they do not work, they do not get paid. What happens if you get sick? Play it safe and wash or disinfect your hands between clients.

For more insights on this topic, see my post entitled "Certified Trainer, but Never Trained Anyone: What to Do," which may be found at Joe-Cannon.com.

Chapter 3

HOW WILL YOU BE PAID?

Let us now talk about how you will be compensated for personal training. Generally, personal trainers tend to either work in a health-club-like setting or are self-employed. We will discuss each separately to give you a better idea what to expect.

Working in a Health Club

If you are working at a health club, there is a good chance that the client will pay the club and you will receive a percentage of that amount. Only rarely do clients pay health-club-based trainers directly. Clubs usually pay every two weeks. You will probably have to keep track of the number of sessions you have with each client and submit that to the club in order to be paid. You may want to use a day planner to help you keep track of the personal training sessions you provide. I like a day planner that shows me one week at a time so that I can see what I have to do during the week. This helps reduce the chances of anything sneaking up on me that might be listed on another page. Payment by health clubs for personal training can vary from place to place, but a couple of scenarios may occur:

1. You get a straight percentage (e.g., 50%) of what you generate
2. Your percentage depends on the number of sessions that you conduct during the week

As a general rule, health clubs pay about 40–65% of the amount collected to the personal trainer. For example, if the client paid the club $300 for 10 sessions with you and the club paid you 50%, you would receive $150 for that client. Usually, health clubs do not automatically pay you the full amount all at once, but pay instead for the number of sessions that you actually execute with that client during the pay period. For example, if you met with the client 3 times during the previous pay period, you would be paid only for those 3 sessions. It is in the club's best interest to do this because it helps to protect the club's members. For example, if the club paid the trainer all of the money up front and the trainer quit, the club—and the client—would be at a loss.

Another popular option in some health clubs is to base the trainer's compensation on the number of sessions he or she performs during the pay period. Under this scenario, trainers who work the most sessions are rewarded for their efforts with a greater percentage of the total amount paid by the client than those trainers who worked fewer sessions. From the club's standpoint, it is in their interest to do this because it stimulates competition among trainers, motivating them to work harder and bringing more money into the club. On the surface, this is a good model, but one possible drawback is that it creates more work for fitness trainers, which may lead to greater frequency of burnout. Some clubs may even do away with the traditional hour-long personal training session and cut it down to 30-minute sessions, allowing a trainer to see more people during the day and thus increasing the amount of money made by the trainer.

Another way that fitness trainers can be compensated is based on their experience. In other words, the more education or certifications you have, the higher your pay rate. Under this system, a trainer who has a BS degree, two certifications, and who has attended regular continuing education seminars might receive more money than someone who only has a college degree and one certification. In the club's eyes, a trainer with more education is more valuable to the organization. Fitness trainers who are also managers may receive higher rates for personal training than non-managers. Moreover, managers may also receive yearly *bonuses* for productive work that they do in their department as well.

Compensation rate for personal training is generally reevaluated at least twice a year. To a reevaluation meeting, bring proof of all of your certifications, awards, and continuing education certificates as well as any degrees that you have. If you have testimonials from clients, bring them as well. The bottom line is that the more valuable you are to the club, the higher your pay rate will be.

Another factor that influences how much you make is whether you receive an hourly rate of pay in addition to personal training compensation. Sometimes the personal training rate you receive may be less because you are a salary-based employee. If you are receiving a salary, the odds are good that you are also getting health insurance benefits. In this instance, the club might cut back on what you get for personal training to compensate for this. In other words, they view you more as an employee and less as a personal trainer. On the other hand, your personal training pay may be higher because your hourly rate is low or you are not working many hours at the club. Perhaps you are only officially working in the club 10 hours a week. Because this probably does not amount to much money, the club might sweeten the deal by giving you a higher percentage of any personal training revenue you generate.

However you are paid, sit down with the club's manager, personal training director, or direct supervisor and have them specifically show you how you will be compensated before beginning to execute training sessions.

Self-Employed Personal Trainers

Self-employed trainers typically charge as much or more per session than gyms charge for training. This is because, as a self-employed personal trainer, you must pay for everything, including equipment, clothing, liability insurance, health insurance, gasoline, and even wear and tear that you put on your car as you travel to people's homes or to other facilities for personal training sessions.

Rates for self-employed trainers vary from place to place. The saying, "Location, location, location!" is really true. Trainers in affluent areas may charge hundreds of dollars for a single session, while those in less well-to-do areas may make much less. Typically, cost ranges from $50-$150 per session. The amount that a trainer makes depends not only on location and education, but also on how well the trainer can market her or himself. Some ways to become more well-known include starting a free walking group for the people in your neighborhood and creating a blog or podcast to demonstrate your knowledge and expertise to others. Social media can also be a valuable tool. Trainers who have knowledge in special areas (e.g., weight loss) can often charge a higher rate as well.

The reimbursement methods for self-employed personal trainers differ significantly from those employed in health clubs, most notably because clients pay them directly. As a self-employed trainer, you have several options: cash, check, or credit card. Unlike trainers who work in a health club setting, self-employed trainers usually receive all of the money up front. They then recharge the client after the number of purchased sessions has been completed. Cash is advantageous because it is immediately usable, but it may be difficult to keep track of who has paid what. Another disadvantage of requesting cash payments is that people do not generally keep large sums of cash on hand. Additionally, unlike other payment methods, if you misplace the money, it is gone. Lastly and most importantly, remember that you must still pay state and federate taxes on all income, including cash.

Another option is to be paid by check. This is a popular method because it is simple and accessible for most people. The disadvantage is that you often have to keep informing the client that their session payments have been depleted and that it is time to renew.

The last option is to set up a merchant account through which you may accept credit card payments. The major advantage here is that a credit card can be charged again immediately when a client uses his or her last session. If you are going to accept credit cards, however there are a few things to keep in mind. First, you need to have a good credit rating. If you have failed to pay loans or bills on time or have declared bankruptcy, you may have difficulty gaining approval for a merchant account.

How to Find Your Credit Rating for Free

By law, the major credit reporting agencies have to provide you with one free report each year. All you have to do is ask for it. You can obtain your reports by going to the website AnnualCreditReport.com. This is a 100% free service that was set up by the three major credit reporting agencies.

Keep in mind that when you accept credit cards, you will probably be required to pay a monthly fee and individual fees on each transaction processed. The monthly fee can fluctuate with the number of credit card transactions you process.

Tips for Getting a Good Credit Rating

1. Pay your bills on time
2. Do not skip payments on credit cards
3. Pay *at least* the monthly minimum on credit card purchases
4. Do not max out your credit cards
5. Avoid signing up for too many credit cards

Several organizations can provide you with a merchant account. Shop around for the one that best suits your needs and check with your local bank for guidance. Searching online for "merchant account" should return information for several companies that provide this service.

Keeping Track of Your Finances

Whether you are self-employed or you work at a health club, you should make an effort to know where your money is going. This will help you see whether you are making or losing money. For self-employed fitness trainers, this is a no-brainer, as you must keep track of money in order to receive tax deductions. Even if you work in a health club, this practice is important. One of the easiest ways to track finances is to get a computer-based money program. All major financial software programs now let you connect online to your bank. This means that the bank will automatically download all bills and deposits you make, and all that you have to do is spend a couple of minutes sorting them into the proper categories. Having the proper categories is the secret to effective money management.

If you pay for some of your business-related items in cash, you can keep track of those as well by using your financial software or by creating a spreadsheet. For example, your spreadsheet might look like this:

Business-Related Cash Expenses

May 2014		
	Business Expense	**Amount**
5/1/14	Ink for printer	$ 19.99
5/5/14	Printer paper	$ 10.00
5/15/14	Financial software	$ 39.99
5/21/14	Book: *Personal Fitness Training Beyond The Basics*	$ 25.95
Total		**$95.93**

Keep all of your business-related cash receipts, tolls, and other documents and add them to the sheet as needed. At the end of the year, print the sheet and give it to your accountant, who can use this information when he or she does your taxes.

Self-employed trainers who travel to people's homes might have a similar spreadsheet for their work-related mileage. For example, the spreadsheet might look something like this:

Business Miles Driven

May 2014	Location Traveled To	Tolls	Round Trip Mileage
10/1/09	Bill Leinhauser	$ 3.00	30
10/16/09	Tim DiFelice	-	25
10/27/09	Paul Coppola	0.75	25
Month Total		**$ 3.75**	**80**

At the end of the year, tally all tolls and miles driven for business. Your accountant can use this information when tax time arrives.

If you go to the bank to make deposits and have more than one source of income, use a different deposit slip for each check. This way, you will know how much each client paid you as well as how much you made from other sources of revenue. You will not know this answer if all deposits are lumped together on the same deposit slip.

Chapter 4

HOW WE MAKE ENERGY

The classic definition of energy is "the ability to do work." Work is anything that you do. For example, reading these words, walking, and lifting weights are all work and require energy. As many know, we make energy from the food we eat. For the most part, energy comes from carbohydrates and fats, while proteins are normally used to a much lesser extent. However, less well-known is the fact that, before we can utilize the energy within the macronutrients (calories), it must first be transformed into a type of energy that our bodies know how to use. For humans, this energy molecule is called **adenosine triphosphate** (ATP). This process is actually very similar to the way that a car works. A car does not run on oil. Rather, the oil has to be refined into gasoline before a vehicle can use it. The same is true for our bodies, which take the raw materials in food and refine them into a "gasoline" that we can use. The process of making energy is technically called **bioenergetics**. This chapter reviews the major ways that we make energy and relates those processes to exercise.

What Does ATP Look Like?

The ATP molecule essentially looks like this:

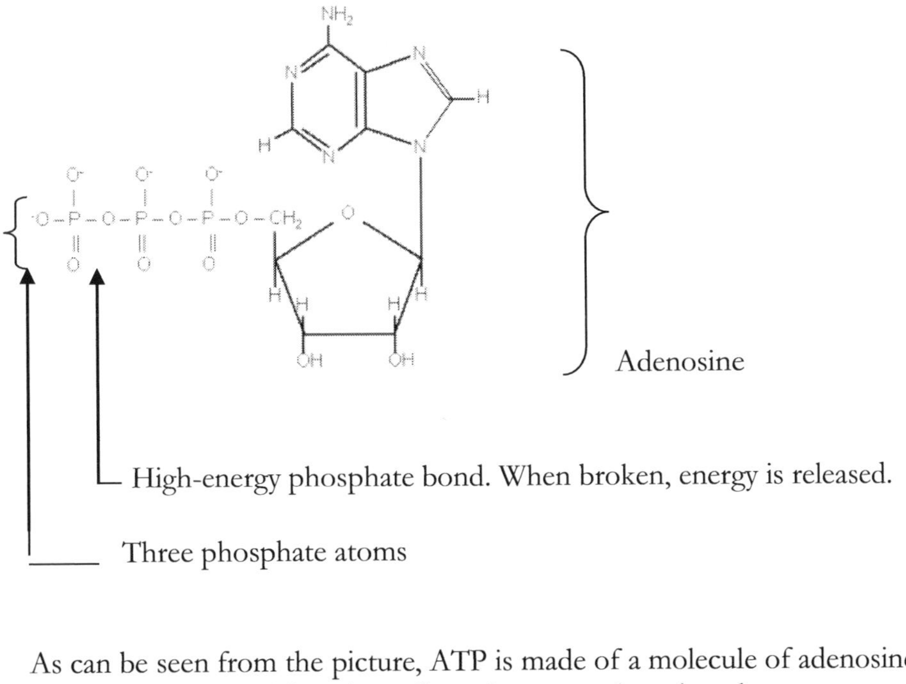

Adenosine

High-energy phosphate bond. When broken, energy is released.

Three phosphate atoms

As can be seen from the picture, ATP is made of a molecule of adenosine (a type to sugar) and three phosphate atoms. The short lines between the phosphate atoms represent energy-containing chemical bonds. The chemical bond attached to the last phosphate is called a **high energy bond.** When this bond is broken, much energy is released. This is the energy that powers all of our activities. The breakdown of ATP is accomplished via an enzyme called an ATPase. When ATP loses its high-energy phosphate, it becomes adenosine diphosphate (ADP). From here, ADP can further break down to adenosine monophosphate (AMP). Neither ADP nor AMP is specifically relevant to the scope of personal training, so they will not be discussed.

Making Energy: The Big Picture

The process of making energy (ATP) is complicated, but there are two primary ways that the body accomplishes this task. One of those ways uses oxygen to make energy and is called the **aerobic energy system**. The other way, which does not need oxygen to work, is called the **anaerobic energy system**. You can think of these energy systems like gears in your car. We have a "gear" inside of us that works at lower intensities of activity and tends to burn a lot of fat. This is the aerobic energy system. The other "gear" that we have works at higher intensities of activity and tends to burn a lot of carbohydrate (sugar). This is the anaerobic energy system. Unlike the gears in your car, however, our gears—aerobic and anaerobic—are always working inside of us. In other words, we are never only burning fat and we are never only burning carbohydrate. For the most part, we are always burning some mixture of fats and carbohydrate to power our energy needs. At lower intensities of activity, we tend to burn greater percentages of fat, while at higher intensities of activity, we tend to burn greater percentages of carbohydrate.

Another important thing to remember is that it is not only the intensity of activity that dictates what we burn for fuel, but also the length of time for which we perform the activity. In other words, if we perform an activity for a long time, we are burning a large percentage of energy from fat to complete that task. If we only perform the activity for a short period of time, on the other hand, carbohydrates (e.g., glucose) supply the bulk of energy needs. For example, reading these words is pretty easy; right now, about 30–40% of the energy that powers this activity comes from carbohydrates. The other 60–70% is coming from fat.[77] This is why you may have read that low-intensity exercise burns fat while high-intensity exercise burns sugar. While this statement is true, some misinterpret it to mean that the best way to burn fat is to do low-intensity exercise. We will address this issue later. For now, let us discuss the aerobic and anaerobic energy systems in greater detail.

The Macronutrients

Food	Calories / Gram[*]
Protein	4
Carbohydrate	4
Fat	9

* There are 28 grams in once ounce.

The Aerobic Energy System

The term aerobic literally means "living in oxygen." One of the most popular names for the aerobic system is the **Krebs cycle**, named in honor of its discoverer, Hans Krebs. Alternative names include the **citric acid cycle** and the **tricarboxylic acid cycle** (TCA cycle). Still another more technical name is **oxidative phosphorylation**. The Krebs cycle is a complex series of chemical reactions that essentially results in energy (ATP) being produced from the breakdown of fat. Thus, people who are trying to lose weight are often counseled to perform aerobic activity because the Krebs cycle uses oxygen to burn fat. The Krebs cycle occurs within the **mitochondria**. Just as our bodies have different organs, the cells of our bodies also have organs called **organelles**, which perform specialized tasks. The mitochondria are one of the many cellular organelles, and one of their main jobs is to burn fat. Biology teachers often call mitochondria the "powerhouses of the cell" because a lot of energy is produced from the breakdown of fat. In reality, mitochondria are like batteries. Just as a battery can produce electrical energy, mitochondria produce biological energy (ATP) and do so in a very similar way to the batteries in your car, cell phone, and other devices. Thus, mitochondria are essentially aerobic, rechargeable, fat-burning batteries.

Human Cell

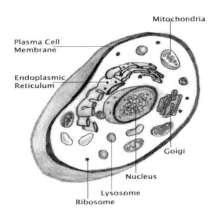

Until now, we have only discussed the Krebs cycle. However, there is another series of chemical reactions that occurs inside the mitochondria. This other chemical reaction series is called the **electron transport chain**, and it is from this mechanism that the battery analogy is derived. The key result of the Krebs cycle and the electron transport chain is that each glucose molecule burned can result in the generation of 38 ATPs.

While a single glucose molecule can produce 38 ATPs, the aerobic breakdown (oxidation) of fat can yield even more energy. Fat is technically called a fatty acid or **triglyceride**. A triglyceride is composed of three long chains of carbon atoms anchored to a glycerol molecule. When fat is broken down, it first enters a chemical reaction called **beta-oxidation,** which chops fat into smaller parts. These parts are transported to the mitochondria with help from a taxicab-like molecule called **carnitine**. The smaller bits of fat then enter the Krebs cycle and electron transport chain, where they produce ATP. Ultimately, hundreds of ATP molecules can be produced from a single triglyceride molecule. As with glycolysis, carbon dioxide (which we exhale) and water are also produced through this process.

When people begin an aerobic exercise training program, the mitochondria in the exercising muscles eventually enlarge and become more numerous. Bigger, more numerous mitochondria can burn more fat. Thus, we would expect to see bigger—and more—mitochondria in the muscles of a triathlete, cyclist, or bodybuilder, as each of these activities has an aerobic component.

Often, those not accustomed to exercise exhaust themselves rather quickly even at low intensities of exercise. One reason for this is that their mitochondria are smaller in size, fewer in number, and less efficient at fat burning. In such instances, the body relies more heavily on burning carbohydrate (glycogen and glucose) anaerobically, which results in the buildup of **lactic acid** (lactate), the substance associated with the burning sensation inside muscles that forces a person to stop exercising. Aerobically trained muscles, on the other hand, use more fat and less glycogen during exercise. Why? It turns out that we need carbohydrates to burn fat. When we run out of carbohydrate, exercise stops. This is why carbohydrates are often called the "rate-limiting fuel." When we work out regularly, our bodies adapt so that they reduce their use of precious glycogen during exercise. In short, we use less carbohydrate and more fat during exercise. While all energy systems are always working inside of us, the aerobic energy system generally begins to contribute significantly to our energy needs during activity lasting longer than 3 minutes.[78]

The Fat-Burn Program

Because low-intensity activities that we can do for long periods of time burn greater percentages of fat, many treadmills feature a "fat-burn" program. Essentially, this program holds people at a relatively low percentage of their maximum heart rate (~60%). While we do indeed burn more fat at lower intensities of activity, this program may not always be ideal for weight loss. For example, walking at 2 mph burns a greater percentage of fat than walking at 3 mph. This also means that sitting burns more fat than standing. Technically, sleeping is the greatest fat-burning activity, with about 70% of the energy coming from fat breakdown. So why do we not lose weight sleeping? Sleeping does not burn many calories. This principle also applies to the fat-burn program. Calories are the key to weight loss (and weight gain).

The fat-burn program does have its advantages. It reduces the risk of injury during exercise and gives people the ability to exercise longer, which in turn results in more calories being used. Thus, for beginners or for those with special needs (e.g., overweight), low-intensity exercise is generally best and safest. The bottom line here is that people should be more focused on burning calories than on burning fat.

The Anaerobic Energy System

The anaerobic energy system basically has two parts: the **ATP/CP system** and **glycolysis**. The ATP/CP system (adenosine triphosphate/creatine phosphate system) is sometimes called the **phosphagen system** because phosphate is common to both compounds. ATP is needed for all activity (exercise and otherwise) to occur. However, we do not store large amounts of ATP in the body. In fact, it is estimated that the body only stores 80–100 grams (3–4 ounces) of ATP at any given moment.[8] Because this is only enough energy for a few seconds of activity, ATP must be constantly made throughout our entire lives.

When exercise demand is very great, **creatine phosphate** is activated. Creatine phosphate (also known as CP or phosphocreatine) is used to replenish ATP at rates faster than other aerobic and anaerobic pathways. In this way, CP acts like a turbocharger for ATP production. During the regeneration process, CP donates its phosphate atom to ADP to reenergize ATP. Then, ATP once again breaks down, releasing the energy that we need. Keep in mind that CP itself cannot provide energy—only by helping reenergize ATP is CP able to contribute to our energy needs. Generally, our cells can store 4–6 times more CP than ATP.[8] This extra energy boost from CP can provide about an extra 10–20 seconds of activity during high-intensity exercise.[8]

$$CP + ADP \rightarrow ATP$$

It is important to remember that the creatine energy source is not being used extensively during activities that the body feels are low-intensity. Thus, in general, CP is not used during activities like walking, hiking, swimming, Yoga, or circuit-style weight training. Rather, CP is used during very heavy weight lifting, sprinting, and other intense activities. Creatine supplementation will further be discussed in the "Questions and Answers" chapter of this book. For more information on creatine and more than 100 other supplements, read my book, *Nutritional Supplements: What Works and Why*, available at Joe-Cannon.com. You may also visit the "Creatine" section of my other site, SupplementClarity.com.

The other part of the anaerobic system is **glycolysis**. Glycolysis refers to a series of chemical reactions in our cells through which ATP (energy) is made via the anaerobic breakdown of carbohydrates. Glycolysis is also sometimes called the **lactic acid system**. This reflects the presence of lactic acid (lactate), a metabolic byproduct formed during glycolysis. The fuel of choice used in glycolysis is the sugar glucose. Glucose is a simple sugar (monosaccharide) that the body prefers to use, which is the reason why it is often called "blood sugar." In fact, some organs of the body (e.g., the brain) must have glucose to function.

Lactic Acid Facts and Myths

Lactic acid is often said to be the cause of muscle burning and fatigue during intense exercise. However, the body does not make lactic acid, but lactate, which is not actually an acid. The burning sensation felt during exercise is currently thought to be due to an increase in hydrogen atoms released as a result of ATP and CP breakdown. As these hydrogen atoms (protons) increase in number, they cause feelings of pain and burning inside the muscles. The rise in hydrogen atoms reduces the pH in the cells, making them more acidic. In turn, this reduces the body's ability to make ATP and inhibits the strength of the myosin/actin cross bridge binding. This ultimately reduces the force production of muscles. With exercise training, however, we get better at dissipating the rise in hydrogen atoms. This is why exercise that once made us fatigued eventually does not do so anymore. Measuring lactate levels can be one way to determine hydrogen atom concentration (e.g., lactate threshold).

It is also a myth that lactate (lactic acid) causes muscle pain the day after exercise (DOMS, Delayed Onset Muscle Soreness). This is because most of the lactate (and hydrogen atoms) has been removed from the cells about an hour or so after exercise. In addition, lactate is not a waste product, but can actually be used for fuel. While most people use the terms "lactic acid" and "lactate" interchangeability, it is important to remember is that they are not the same thing.[186]

During glycolysis, glucose is sent through a series of chemical reactions, which results in the creation of ATP (energy). Specifically, 2 ATPs can be made per glucose molecule (3 ATPs if we use glycogen). In addition, a byproduct called **pyruvate** is made. Pyruvate, in turn, has the opportunity to be converted into a similar molecule called lactate ("lactic acid"). Pyruvate may take another path as well. In the case where exercise is easy enough that sufficient oxygen is present, pyruvate does not become lactate, but is transported to the mitochondria and converted into another compound called acetyl coenzyme A, which helps produce even more ATPs via the Krebs cycle. This alternative route is sometimes called aerobic glycolysis because oxygen is used to help further metabolize pyruvate to make more ATP molecules. Those struggling with this concept and wondering which aspect of glycolysis—aerobic or anaerobic—occurs during different types of activities may remember that, during high-intensity activities (when ATP must be made rapidly), anaerobic glycolysis predominates. During low-intensity activities (when ATP does not need to be made as quickly), aerobic glycolysis and the Krebs cycle are more likely to occur. Generally speaking, glycolysis contributes significantly to our energy needs during exercise lasting 2–3 minutes.[78] After that, the aerobic energy system starts to prevail.

It is important for fitness professionals to understand that when carbohydrates are eaten, they are chemically rearranged into glucose. Glucose, in turn, is either used immediately or stored in the body in the form of another molecule called **glycogen**. When needed, glycogen is broken down into glucose, which then enters cells to be made into energy (ATP). Thus, glucose and glycogen are basically the same thing. The formation of glycogen from glucose is called **glycogenesis**. Conversely, the breakdown of glycogen to form glucose is called **glucogenolysis**. One major difference between glycolysis and the Krebs cycle is that glycolysis occurs inside the watery cytoplasm of the cells. The Krebs cycle, on the other hand, occurs in the mitochondria, which float within the cytoplasm.

The Lactate Threshold

The lactate threshold is the point during exercise when lactate levels begin to rise dramatically in the blood. In other words, it is the moment when one begins to rely heavily upon anaerobic energy systems to sustain exercise. Hydrogen atoms begin to accumulate significantly at this point as well. Another name for this point is **lactate inflection point** (LIP). For those accustomed to exercise, this threshold is usually reached at about 70–80% Karvonen HR max (~70–80% VO2max), while for untrained people, it is typically reached and at ~50–60% Karvonen HR max.[78] If exercise continues to increase beyond this point, another inflection point occurs at which lactate levels rise even further. This second threshold is called the **Onset of Blood Lactate Accumulation** (OBLA). Here, there is an even greater accumulation of lactate and hydrogen atoms in the blood. According to some, OBLA corresponds with the body's greater reliance on type II muscle fibers, which are recruited in greater numbers to help sustain the exercise intensity.[78]

For athletes, training at intensities close to or at lactate threshold or OBLA may help the body better deal with lactate clearance and push back the intensities at which these thresholds occur. In theory, this may help athletes exercise at higher intensities without facing significant muscle burning and fatigue. That said, most people who hire personal trainers do not need to worry about this. For the majority of people, moderate-intensity exercise of 20–60 minutes most days of the week suits their needs well.

Exercise Intensity and Duration: Distinguishing between Aerobic and Anaerobic

Exercise Intensity & Duration	Energy System Used
High-Intensity, Short-Lasting	Primarily anaerobic
Low-Intensity, Long-Lasting	Primarily aerobic

Which Sports Use Which Energy System?

In general, it can be said that any activity that one can perform for a long period of time uses the aerobic energy system to a greater degree than the anaerobic system. Conversely, any activity that one can only perform for a short period of time primarily utilizes the anaerobic system. The following are some examples of activities and the energy systems that they primarily use:[24]

ATP/CP System (mostly)	ATP/CP & Glycolysis	Glycolysis (mostly)	Glycolysis & Krebs cycle	Krebs Cycle (mostly)
100 m sprint	200 m sprint	400 m sprint	800 m sprint	Triathlon
1RM lift	Baseball homerun	Tennis	Boxing	Marathon
Diving	Basketball	100 m swim	Rugby	Jogging
Jumping	Ice hockey sprint	Soccer	1 mile run	Cross country skiing

It should be stressed that, in reality, it is the fitness level of the person that really determines which energy system is used during exercise. In other words, it is possible for an activity that is traditionally considered aerobic to be perceived by an untrained person to be anaerobic. Some people may be so unfit (due to old age, sarcopenia, disease, and other conditions) that walking a few yards overwhelms the aerobic system. In such instances, the person relies heavily upon the anaerobic energy system. This, in turn, causes the person to run out of steam sooner than expected. Since most people who hire trainers are beginners, this must be considered during training.

Protein Use and Exercise

As a general rule, protein contributes about 2–10% of our energy needs, although others estimate its rate of breakdown can be as much as 20% in some extreme instances.[86] Protein use is likely to be elevated during long-lasting exercise (e.g., a marathon), especially in people with poor diets. Two key nutrients that help us preserve protein are calories and carbohydrates, which must be consumed in adequate quantities. In the absence of enough calories (e.g., dieting), protein may be broken down to help create energy to make up for what is no longer being consumed. Specifically, protein can be transformed into glucose via **gluconeogenesis**. The glucose produced can be used for energy. Athletes sometimes supplement with branch chain amino acids (BCAA) because they can be burned for energy inside muscle cells.[38] The BCAAs are leucine, isoleucine, and valine. Other studies suggest that these amino acids may help reduce fatigue during exercise.[38] Less well known to people is the role that carbohydrates play in helping to preserve muscle tissue. Carbohydrates can help prevent protein from being broken down just as BCAA supplements might. For those on a budget, carbohydrates may be a cheaper alternative.

Sometimes people report that they smell like ammonia after working out. This often happens in those who are also eating a low-carbohydrate/high-protein diet. Remember that carbohydrates help protect protein from being used for fuel. In the absence of enough carbohydrates, the body starts to break down the amino acids in protein to maintain its energy needs. In the process, ammonia is produced and sweated out of the pores of the body. This is an example of gluconeogenesis. Increasing carbohydrate intake or drinking more water should help correct this problem.

What Happens after Exercise?

After the cessation of exercise, the energy that has been expended must be replaced. For example, lactate that accumulates during exercise can be transformed into glucose and stored as glycogen via a series of chemical reactions called the Cori Cycle. It is interesting to note that the energy expended via the anaerobic energy systems are reenergized via the aerobic energy system. More specifically, after exercise, people continue to breathe more deeply than normal for a period of time. The extra oxygen consumed helps the aerobic system replenish the energy stores used during anaerobic exercise. This is sometimes called "oxygen debt." A more descriptive term for this is **excessive postexercise oxygen consumption** (EPOC). Another way of thinking about this is to consider the fact that metabolic rate remains elevated after exercise has stopped. Both aerobic and anaerobic exercise elevates EPOC, but which does so the most? This will be addressed in the "Question and Answer" chapter of this book.

Practical Applications

Fitness professionals should have a working knowledge of energy systems because this can help them train their clients according to their individual needs and goals. Remember, the body responds specifically to the exercise demands placed upon it (this is referred to as the "SAID Principle"). For example, those who want to improve sprinting performance should focus on developing their anaerobic energy systems. Many sports involve various combinations of all energy systems, so the job of the trainer is to determine the ideal mix for the client. Whatever the person's goal, it is wise to begin the program at a low intensity and progress to the desired level of fitness over time.

Chapter 5

ANATOMY AND PHYSIOLOGY

The Planes of the Body

Movement can occur in different orientations or planes. The planes in which movement can occur are the sagittal plane, the frontal plane, and transverse plane.

Sagittal plane. Imagine a vertical line going through the body and breaking it up into both left and right sides. This is the sagittal plane.

Frontal plane. Imagine a line cutting the body into two parts—front and back. This is the frontal plane.

Transverse plane. In this plane, a line divides the person into an upper and lower part. A visual analogy of this would be a magician who "saws" a lady in half.

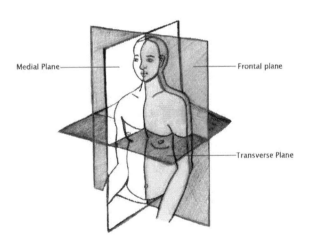

It is important to remember that, while three planes of movement are usually discussed, human movement patterns in everyday life sometimes involve 2 or more planes at once. This gives rise to the term **triplanar,** which refers to movements that occur in real life. This notion has increased the popularity of the term "functional" in the fitness world. **Functional movement patterns** are those that mimic what a person does in the real world. For example, getting up from the floor is more functional than using the leg press machine. In a pure sense, functional exercises attempt to train movement patterns in addition to muscles.

Common Anatomy Terms

Medial. Medial refers to being close to the midline of the body. If you were performing internal shoulder rotation, you would be rotating your arm medially, or toward the body.

Lateral. Lateral refers to being farther away from the body. It also refers to movement away from the midline of the body. If you were doing external shoulder rotation, you would be moving your arm laterally from the body.

Proximal. Proximal refers to being close to a reference point or the midline of the body. For example, the humerus is more proximal to the shoulder than the radius bone.

Distal. Distal refers to something being situated far from its point of origin or reference point. For example, the foot is more distal from the head than is the nose.

Pronation. This is used to describe the action of turning your hand such that your that the palm is facing downward. For example, if you perform a reverse biceps curl, you do so with your hands in the pronated position. With respect to the feet, pronation occurs when the foot is oriented such that the inner portion of the foot is rotated inward. The prone position also occurs when you lay face down.

Supination. This is used to describe the action of rotating your hands so that your palms are facing up. The biceps is responsible for supination, which this is why some supinate their hands as they lift dumbbells. The thought behind this practice is that combining both actions of the biceps (elbow flexion and supination) would stimulate the biceps to grow more.

Superior. This term usually refers to being above a reference point. For example, the head is more superior to the heart than the feet. The superior vena cava returns blood to the heart from the upper portion of the body.

Inferior. Inferior refers to being below a reference point. For example, the femur bone is inferior to the ribs. The inferior vena cava returns blood to the heart from the lower portions of the body.

Anterior. This term refers to being in front or before the body, an organ, or a reference point. For example, the anterior deltoid composes the front portion of the deltoid muscle group. Anterior is the opposite of posterior.

Posterior. This refers to being behind a reference point or located toward the rear. It is the opposite of anterior. For example, the back of the shoulder is often referred to as the posterior deltoid.

Plantarflexion. This term usually refers to the foot and is used when the foot is bent such that the toes are pointing straight ahead. A dancer on her tippy toes reflects this action.

Dorsiflexion. This term usually refers to the foot and is used when the foot is bent such that the toes are brought close to the body. Walking on your heels requires you to dorsiflex your feet.

Tissues of the Body

A **tissue** is a group of cells that performs a specific function. Generally speaking, four groups of tissues are usually discussed: epithelial tissue, nerve tissue, connective tissue, and muscle tissue.

Epithelial tissue is comprised of single cell layers of tissue that serve many different functions. For example, epithelial cells line the insides of the blood vessels (i.e., endothelial cells), where they ensure proper, turbulence-free movement of blood, while epithelial cells on the surface of the skin act as a barrier between you and the outside environment.

Nerve tissue conducts electrical impulses between the brain and the rest of the body.

Connective tissue serves a number of purposes such as forming tendons and ligaments as well as providing an overall structural framework to the body. Bone, blood, and fat are all connective tissues. Another connective tissue called cartilage can also act as a shock absorber between bones.

Muscle tissue allows us to not only interact with the outside environment, but to survive as well. Muscle tissue can be subdivided into three types: smooth muscle, cardiac muscle, and skeletal muscle. **Smooth muscle** lines blood vessels and allows them to expand and contract when needed. **Cardiac muscle** is heart muscle. One of the main differences of cardiac muscle and others is that its contraction is involuntary. In other words, we do not have to think about making the heart contract. This is good news—if we had to think in order to get the heart to contract, none of us would live for very long! **Skeletal muscle** is the type that is usually of most interest to fitness professionals. It is called "skeletal" because, for the most part, it is attached to the skeleton (e.g., in the biceps, quadriceps, and other muscle groups).

Organs are specialized tissues that perform specific tasks. For example, the heart, kidneys, brain, skin, and lungs are all organs. A **gland** is a specialized type of organ that produces a substance (e.g., a hormone) that is released into the blood or body cavity. Generally, two types of glands are recognized: exocrine glands and endocrine glands. **Exocrine glands** secrete substances into a duct or passageway that is close to where it is located. Examples of an exocrine gland include mammary glands, sweat glands, and salivary glands. **Endocrine glands**, on the other hand, generally secrete substances (e.g., hormones) into the blood, where they can then travel far from their place of origin. For example, the beta cells of the pancreas make the hormone insulin, which travels through the blood and helps cells process sugar (glucose) and amino acids.

Examples of Endocrine Glands and the Hormones They Produce

Gland	Selected Hormone Made	Function
Adrenal glands	Adrenaline (epinephrine)	Fight or flight response
Pineal gland	Melatonin	Sleep
Pituitary gland	Growth hormone	Growth and various other functions
Thyroid gland	Thyroid hormone	Regulates metabolism
Pancreas	Insulin and glucagon	Decreases and increases blood sugar respectively
Kidneys	Erythropoietin (EPO)	Makes red blood cells
Liver	Insulin-like growth factors (IGFs)	Various functions
Skin	Vitamin D	Improves calcium absorption
Testes	Testosterone	Muscle growth and other functions

Two other examples of endocrine glands that are of particular interest to fitness professionals are fat cells and the stomach. Fat cells (adipose cells) secrete a hormone called **leptin,** which plays a role in eating. When leptin levels are high (e.g., after eating), the hormone sends a signal that we are full. When leptin levels are low, the signal is that we are hungry.[49]Another hormone is **ghrelin**, which is made in the stomach. High levels of ghrelin stimulate appetite, while low levels reduce appetite.[50] It is important to remember that, while leptin and ghrelin play roles in eating and gaining weight, they are not the only players in the game. People eat for a variety of reasons. Fitness professionals should ask for peer-reviewed evidence for any nutritional supplement touted to promote weight loss by blocking or inhibiting either of these hormones.

Connective Tissue and Cartilage

Connective tissue is a general term for diverse tissues that serve many different functions. Blood, bone, tendons, and cartilage are all examples of connective tissues that help the body function properly. Cartilage is one of the most prevalent connective tissues in the body, helping to form joints, ribs, tendons, ligaments, and ears. Because of its dense nature, cartilage is able to sustain great forces without being damaged, making it perfect for the ends of long bones of the body, where it helps reduce friction and serves as a shock absorber. In the presence of **osteoarthritis**, this cartilage is damaged, which results in pain as bones grind together. Cartilage is avascular, which means that it has no direct blood supply. For this reason, tendons and ligaments take a long time to heal after they are injured. One component of cartilage that helps give the tissue its strength is chondroitin sulfate. Chondroitin sulfate is also marketed as a dietary supplement to help osteoarthritis.[38] Evidence for this supplement helping arthritis, though, is uncertain.[38]

Two types of cartilage are generally discussed: fibrous cartilage and hyaline cartilage. **Fibrous cartilage** is sturdy and found in tendons and ligaments as well as in the disks of the spinal cord. Conversely, **hyaline cartilage** is found in areas like the trachea (i.e., the wind pipe) and at the ends of the long bones of the body (e.g., femur). The hyaline cartilage found at the ends of bones is often called **articular cartilage** or joint cartilage (articular means joint). This is the cartilage worn away in osteoarthritis.

Tendons

A tendon is a tough band of connective tissue (mostly collagen) that usually connects muscles to bones. When muscles are worked, the force of that activity is transmitted from the muscles to the tendons, which in turn pull on the bone. This is why it is possible for resistance training to strengthen bones and help offset osteoporosis. In other words, as you strengthen muscles, you also strengthen bones.

At the point where the tendon and muscle come together (called the myotendinous junction) is a specialized sensor called the **Golgi tendon organ** (GTO). The GTO monitors force production by the muscle. If the GTO senses that the muscle is producing so much force that it or the tendon might be damaged, the GTO activates. When this happens, the GTO relaxes the muscle. In extreme instances, the GTO may also cause the contraction of the antagonistic muscle to further help reduce injury. You can think of the GTO as a safety mechanism that protects the body from harm.

Many people outside of fitness are unaware of the GTO. This, coupled with the desire to lift heavy weights, has the potential to lead to serious injury. For example, consider a novice who is performing very heavy bench presses without a spotter. This person lifts so much weight that the GTO activates. The GTO "thinks" that an injury to the muscle or tendon is about to occur—it does not "know" that the person has 300 pounds suspended above his or her body. In this situation, the muscle relaxes and the barbell falls onto the person, causing serious and possibly life-threatening injury. This is why it is always recommended that people have a spotter when lifting weights. Fortunately, by employing **progressive overload resistance training**, muscles, tendons, and ligaments all grow stronger over time which resets the point at which the GTO activates. This is why it is possible for some people to lift tremendous amounts of weight.

Muscle Spindles

Related to the GTO is another type of receptor called the **muscle spindle**. Muscle spindles reside within the muscle and relay information about the length of the and about how fast the muscle changes its length. When the muscle spindles sense that a muscle is stretching too quickly, they send a signal to the CNS, which in turn relays a signal back to the muscle to contract. In this way, muscle spindles protect muscles from being stretched too far or too rapidly.

With respect to stretching, this is why it is recommended that a person not stretch too quickly or to the point of pain. Doing so activates the muscle spindles, which contract the muscle, and this defeats the purpose of stretching. This phenomenon is sometimes called the "stretch reflex."

Muscle spindles are essentially modified muscle fibers and are sometimes called **intrafusal fibers** to differentiate them from the **extrafusal muscle fibers,** also known as slow- and fast-twitch fibers). Both muscle spindles and GTOs are referred to as **proprioceptors**, specialized sensory receptors that monitor and relay information about motion or body position.

Tendon placement can also play a role in how strong a person is or can be. Thus, where a tendon attaches to the bone can dictate how much force the muscle associated with that tendon can produce. This might play a role in how big muscles have the potential to become via strength training. Tendon placement is genetically predetermined and cannot be altered by training.

Ligaments

Like tendons, ligaments are also made of tough connective tissue composed mostly of collagen. Ligaments connect the bones together. When one bone is connected to another, a joint is formed.

Joints

A joint is formed when two bones come together. Another term for joint is **articulation.** The disorder known as arthritis is one that affects the joints. **Osteoarthritis** (abbreviated as OA or DJD), the most common form of arthritis, occurs when the cartilage cushion between joints wears away. The type called **rheumatoid arthritis** (abbreviated RA), on the other hand, occurs because of an autoimmune disorder whereby the immune system attacks the joints of the body, causing inflammation and pain.

There are different joints of the body, and each type serves different purposes and has a different range of motion (ROM). The shape of bones, the toughness or tightness of ligaments, and even the arrangement of muscles around a joint can impact the joint's ROM. Some people claim to be "double jointed." Often, this situation is caused by ligaments that are not as tight as "normal" joints. A dislocation (luxation) can occur when one of the bones forming a joint is out of place. A subluxation is a partial or incomplete dislocation. Common signs of a dislocation can include swelling, pain, or loss of motion in the joint following an activity.[133] A synovial joint is one of the most common types, and it is given its name because of the synovial membrane that covers the joint. The synovial membrane makes a fluid called synovial fluid, which helps reduce friction. The shoulder, wrist, knee, and elbow all contain synovial joints.

The Human Skeleton

The skeleton can be divided into two parts: the axial skeleton and the appendicular skeleton. The **axial skeleton** is composed of the skull, vertebral column, sternum, and ribs. *The appendicular skeleton* is composed of the long bones of the upper and lower body (humerus, radius, ulna, femur, fibula, and tibia) as well as the scapula, clavicle, and pelvis.

Human Skeleton Anterior View

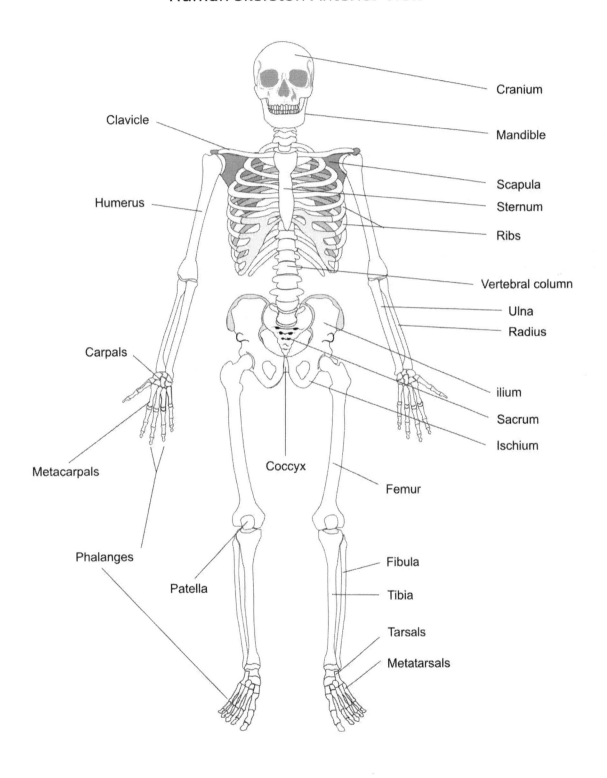

Cranium

Mandible

Clavicle

Scapula

Sternum

Humerus

Ribs

Vertebral column

Ulna

Radius

Carpals

ilium

Sacrum

Ischium

Metacarpals

Coccyx

Femur

Phalanges

Fibula

Patella

Tibia

Tarsals

Metatarsals

33

Human Skeleton Posterior View

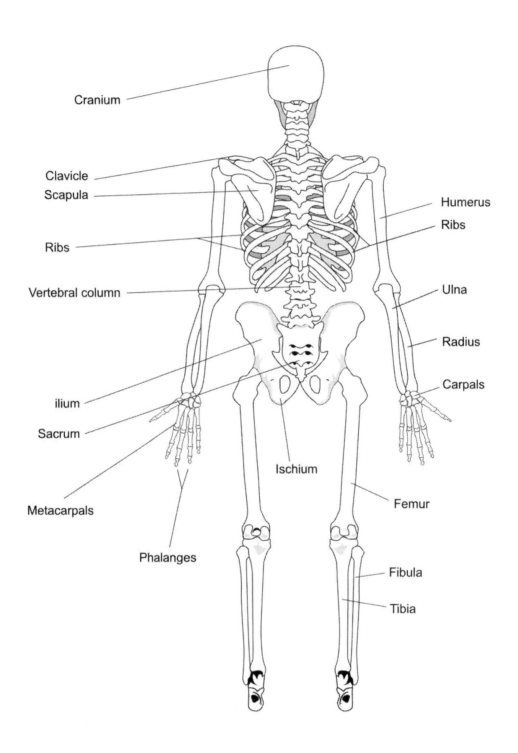

Cranium

Clavicle

Scapula

Ribs

Vertebral column

ilium

Sacrum

Metacarpals

Phalanges

Humerus

Ribs

Ulna

Radius

Carpals

Ischium

Femur

Fibula

Tibia

The Spinal Column

From top to bottom, the major sections of the spinal (vertebral) column are called cervical, thoracic, lumbar, sacral, and coccygeal. There are 7 **cervical vertebrae** (numbered C1 to C7); 12 **thoracic vertebrae** (numbered T1 to T12); 5 **lumbar vertebrae** (numbered L1 to L5); 5 **sacral vertebrae** (numbered S1 to S5) and 3–5 fused bones in the **coccygeal** area. The coccygeal area (also called coccyx) is sometimes called the "tailbone" because of the thought that it is a leftover from an earlier stage of evolution. It is estimated that more than 90% of low back problems occur in the lumbar spine, specifically in the area from L5–S1 (between the 5th lumbar vertebrae and the 1st sacral vertebrae).

Bone

There are 206 bones in the adult human body and they make up about 20% of the body weight of an adult. Besides providing "scaffolding" for the body, bones also act as a reservoir for minerals (e.g., calcium) if needed. The bone marrow is also where red blood cells (RBCs) are formed.[24] Small bones in our ears are also primarily responsible for our ability to hear. Bone is actually a living tissue that is constantly undergoing growth, repair, and degradation processes. Bone can be divided into two forms: cortical bone and trabecular bone. **Cortical bone** is dense and compact and forms the hard, outer shell of bone. **Trabecular bone** (also called cancellous bone or spongy bone) is softer and is found inside bone, but it also adds to bone strength.

There are four types of bones in the body: long, short, flat, and irregularly-shaped bones. The bone shaft of long bones is called the **diaphysis**, while the ends of these bones are called the **epiphysis**. It is at the ends of long bones (epiphysis) that long bones grow longer. These regions are called the **epiphysial plates** (growth plates). Growth plate damage is often cited as a reason to dissuade kids from lifting weights. While damage is certainly possible, especially with maximal and/or overhead lifts, research also finds that supervised resistance training can actually help reduce injuries in adolescents.[77]

The process of bone formation is called **osteogenesis** ("osteo" means "bone"). Bone growth and repair is complex, and three types of cells are usually described: osteoblasts, osteocytes, and osteoclasts. **Osteoblasts** are essentially baby bone cells. Osteoblast cells begin bone formation by making several proteins and related compounds including collagen, calcium carbonate, and calcium phosphate. These become the **matrix** of bone. Eventually, the matrix hardens, giving bone its strength. Because the matrix of bone is related to its strength, health professionals often discuss a concept called **bone mineral density** (BMD). The greater the BMD, the stronger the bone is.

Osteoblast cells eventually become mature bone cells called **osteocytes**. Cells called **osteoclasts** degrade bone. As osteoclasts degrade bone, its minerals (e.g., calcium) are released for the body to use if adequate nutrients are not consumed in the diet. Ultimately, this process can lead to bone being degraded faster than it can be made, resulting in a loss of BMD. Eventually, this process can make bones porous and weak, leading to osteoporosis. This is why an unhealthy diet is partially linked to osteoporosis. Fortunately, because muscles are attached to the bones, it is possible for strength training to help counteract osteoporosis. It is important for fitness professionals to remember that osteoporosis is not simply a condition that affects elderly people. Long-term bed rest, various diseases, and lack of physical activity can all lead to reduced bone density. Men can develop osteoporosis as well as women. Some evidence hints that the greatest rate of bone loss occurs within the first seven weeks of no physical activity.[41]

Chapter 6

MUSCLE PHYSIOLOGY

The human body has over 600 skeletal muscles. Interestingly, muscles are only able to pull—no muscle can push anything. It is only because of the intricate interactions between different muscles and their associated bones that we are able to perform pushing actions. This chapter deals with various issues related to muscle physiology that are important for fitness professionals to understand. This chapter is by no means comprehensive—people have devoted their entire lives to discovering how muscles work, and many fine books have been written solely on this topic. The goal of this section is simply to cut to the chase and to provide the fitness professional with relevant information without going into the nitty-gritty details that do not typically arise in conversation with the general public.

Human Muscles Anterior View

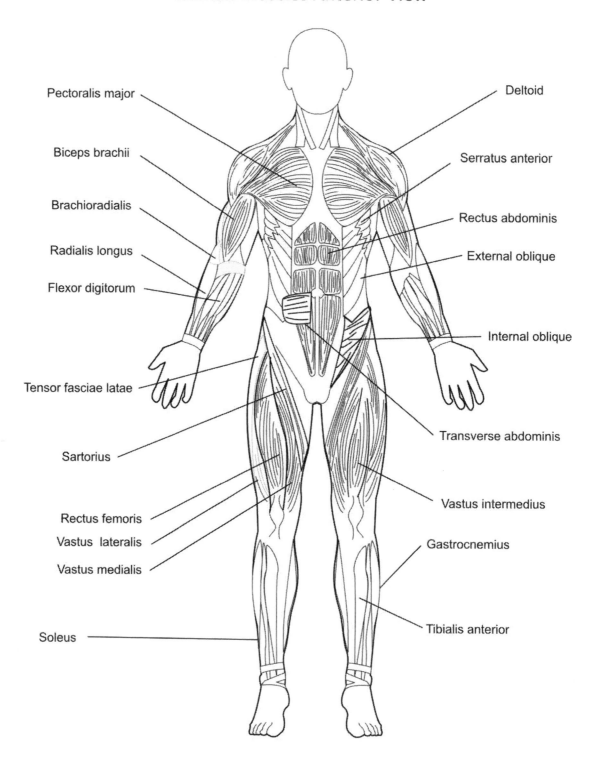

Pectoralis major

Biceps brachii

Brachioradialis

Radialis longus

Flexor digitorum

Tensor fasciae latae

Sartorius

Rectus femoris

Vastus lateralis

Vastus medialis

Soleus

Deltoid

Serratus anterior

Rectus abdominis

External oblique

Internal oblique

Transverse abdominis

Vastus intermedius

Gastrocnemius

Tibialis anterior

Human Muscles Posterior View

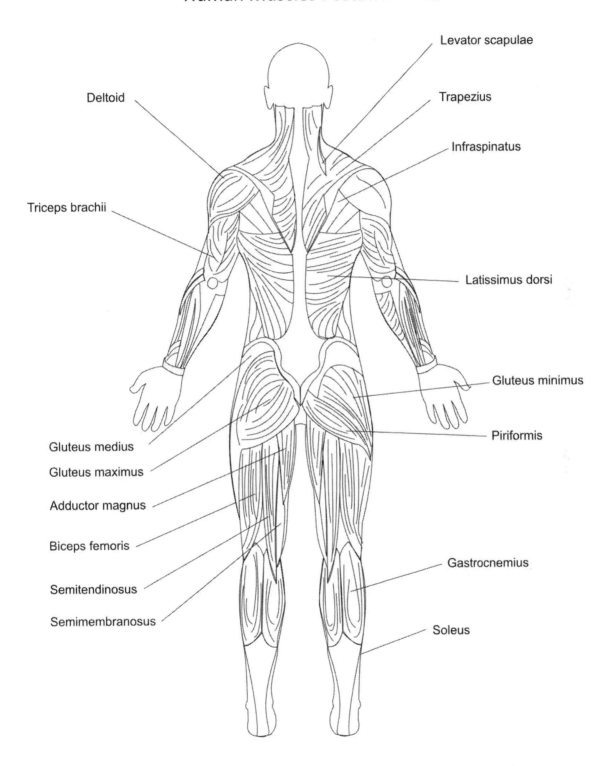

Levator scapulae

Deltoid

Trapezius

Infraspinatus

Triceps brachii

Latissimus dorsi

Gluteus minimus

Piriformis

Gluteus medius

Gluteus maximus

Adductor magnus

Biceps femoris

Gastrocnemius

Semitendinosus

Semimembranosus

Soleus

Basic Muscle Physiology

Since fitness professionals deal with muscles, it is important that they have a grasp of how muscles work. Let us now discuss the basic structure of a muscle fiber. Muscles are made of muscle fibers, also called muscle cells. As mentioned previously, muscles are attached to bones by way of tendons. If you could pull a muscle cell out of the body, you would see that it is covered by a connective tissue called the **epimysium**. In fact, tendons are basically extensions of the epimysium that reach out and grab onto bones. Looking more deeply into a muscle you would see that the fibers are bundled into groups called **fascicles**, which are covered by connective tissue called the **perimysium.** Each muscle fiber that makes up a fascicle is further covered by connective tissue called **endomysium.**[24] It is important to remember that each connective tissue layer—epimysium, perimysium, and endomysium—is basically an extension of the tendon.[78] Thus, when a muscle produces force, that force is transmitted back to the tendon, which then pulls on the bone. This is how strength training the muscles also strengthens bone. The membrane surrounding each muscle fiber is called the **sarcolemma.**[24]

As mentioned previously, a fascicle is a group of muscle fibers (muscle cells). If you could pull out one of the fibers that make up a fascicle, you would see that the fiber is made up of even smaller units called **myofibrils**.[78] Myofibrils are composed of a variety of smaller myofilament proteins. Two of these proteins are myosin and actin. While **myosin** is a thick protein, **actin** is a thinner protein. These myosin and actin proteins are stacked or layered on top of one another inside myofibrils, giving the fibers a striped appearance and making up the force-generating functional unit of muscle contraction—the **sarcomere**. When a muscle contracts, the sarcomeres that compose the muscle fiber are the components that actually contract. During the contraction process, actin and myosin protein filaments slide over each other. This leads us into the next topic—the sliding filament theory of muscle contraction.

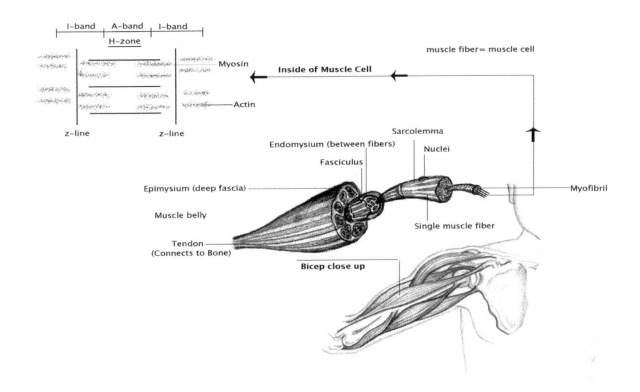

The Sliding Filament Theory

The process that best describes how our muscles function is referred to as the **sliding filament theory** of muscle contraction, which was first postulated in the 1950s.[29,41] According to this theory, the actin and myosin proteins (myofilaments) are contained within **sarcomeres**, which are the basic units of muscle contraction. Muscle cells are made up of many sarcomeres, which are layered or stacked on top of each other.

When stimulated to contract, actin and myosin filaments literally slide over each other as a muscle is worked. More specifically, the thin actin proteins are pulled by the thick myosin proteins in a "ratcheting" motion. This is made possible because the myosin proteins have globular heads jutting from them that reach over to make contact with actin proteins. You can visualize these myosin globular heads as using the image of the head of a golf club. They form a bridge, called a **cross bridge**, that travels across from the myosin protein to the actin proteins. When stimulated by nerve impulses, the globular head of the myosin cross bridge attaches to its corresponding attachment site on the actin protein and pulls it. It then releases and reattaches itself to another attachment site along the actin protein and pulls again. As this ratcheting process (called **cross bridge cycling**) continues, the muscle shortens and contracts, generating the force needed to perform work such as standing up, walking, or curling a barbell.

The energy that powers the cross bridge on myosin to pull the actin filaments during muscle contraction is supplied by ATP. Myosin proteins contain an enzyme called a myosin ATPase, which breaks down ATP, releasing the energy needed for cross bridge cycling to occur.[22] It is interesting to note that ATP does not directly cause myosin to pull actin. Rather, ATP is needed for the myosin cross bridge to detach from its attachment site on the actin filament. After it detaches from one site, it is able to reattach to another site and pull actin once again.

Can We Run Out of ATP?

While exhaustive exercise may diminish ATP levels for a short time, they are never depleted entirely. The body is very good at continually producing ATP through both its aerobic and anaerobic energy systems. In fact, if we were not able to make ATP, we would die! "Rigor mortis," one of the earliest signs of death, occurs when the muscles become rigid and may no longer be easily moved. This phenomenon is due to the inability of the body to produce ATP any longer. In the absence of ATP, the myosin cross bridges are basically "frozen" to the actin filaments, causing the rigid appearance indicative of rigor mortis.

Recall that we have different types of muscle fibers—type I (slow-twitch) and type II (fast-twitch). It turns out that fast-twitch fibers have a myosin ATPase enzyme that breaks down ATP faster than slow-twitch fibers.[41] The more quickly ATP can be broken down, the more quickly cross bridge cycling can occur, allowing the muscle to contract more rapidly. This is the origin of the name, "fast-twitch" muscle fibers.

Obviously, the sliding filament theory is a lot more complicated than what has been described here. In fact, we still call it a "theory" because no one has ever seen living tissue contract at the molecular level.

The Brain/Muscle Connection

The fact that we must think before skeletal muscle does anything means that there is a connection between muscles and the brain. Let us now talk about that connection and how it works.

The process that describes how a nerve impulse induces a muscle contraction is referred to as **excitation-contraction coupling** because it couples or connects the excitatory (stimulating) signals of the nervous system with the contracting muscles. When we make a conscious decision to move a muscle, the impulse starts in the brain in an area called the **primary motor area.** It is here that an excitatory brain chemical called a neurotransmitter (such as acetylcholine) is released from a brain cell called a neuron to travel over to another neuron. Ultimately, this generates a nerve impulse (called an **action potential**). This process continues from cell to cell until the signal reaches the muscle. It is important to note that the stimulus needed to produce a nerve impulse must be of sufficient strength before an impulse is created. This makes sense—otherwise, any stimulus that we encounter during the day could lead to muscle contractions or other involuntary reactions. Only after an impulse crosses this threshold is an action potential generated.

The regeneration of the nerve signals from one brain cell to another is accomplished as the neurotransmitter alters the concentration of sodium and potassium (**electrolytes**) within cells. More specifically, when the neurotransmitter reaches another cell, it causes potassium to temporarily leave the cell, while at the same time allowing sodium to temporarily rush into the cell. The effect of this is that the electrical nature of the cell momentarily transforms from electrically positive to electrically negative. This temporary electrical depolarization of cells allows nervous impulses to travel throughout the body.

When the nerve impulse reaches the muscle, it first makes contact with the gap or space between the nerve cell and muscle cell (called the **neuromuscular junction**). From here, it travels across that space to the muscle cell. Upon reaching the muscle cell, the impulse makes contact with the muscle cell membrane (**sarcolemma**), where it again causes alterations in the concentration of sodium and potassium. In other words, sodium enters the cell while potassium exits. This process further spreads the impulse over the muscle cell in a manner similar to the way that water spreads out over a table. The action potential (nerve impulse) then travels down into the muscle cell by way of channels called the transverse tubules (**T-tubules**). This stimulates a portion of the cell called the **sarcoplasmic reticulum** (SR), which contains calcium. When stimulated by the nerve impulse, the sarcoplasmic reticulum releases calcium into the cell.

Before we go any further, let us introduce two additional muscle proteins called **troponin** and **tropomyosin**, which sit on the actin protein molecule and are important for regulating how actin and myosin interact. Essentially, troponin sits on top of tropomyosin, blocking the myosin attachment site when the muscle is relaxed. When calcium is released from the sarcoplasmic reticulum, it diffuses through the cell and makes contact with troponin. This causes the troponin to shift its position and, in doing so, moves tropomyosin out of the way, revealing the actin attachment sites. This creates space for the myosin cross bridges to bind, facilitating muscle contraction.

Obviously, it would not be good for muscles to constantly contract, so there must be a way for muscles to relax. Remember that the sarcoplasmic reticulum releases calcium into the cell. The SR has cellular pumps that remove calcium from the cell and return it to its storage site. As calcium levels fall within the cell, the troponin-tropomyosin complex returns to its resting state, once again blocking the attachment sites on actin and causing muscles to relax.

What Are Motor Units?

Muscle fibers (muscle cells) are stimulated by nerves. The nerves that stimulate movement are called motor nerves or motor neurons. They are also sometimes called **alpha motor neurons**. A **motor unit** refers to a motor neuron (brain cell or nerve) and all of the muscle cells that it directly stimulates.[30] The motor nerves send electrochemical signals from the brain down the spinal column, and those signals eventually reach muscle cells. In this way, the brain tells a muscle to contract.

When a motor unit is stimulated, all of its associated muscle fibers contract. Different muscles can have different numbers of motor units. In general, the more precise the movement, the fewer muscle fibers are stimulated by a single motor unit. For example, the eye muscles may have very few muscle fibers associated with a motor unit, while a biceps muscle may have thousands of fibers per unit. Most muscles have hundreds to thousands of motor units associated with them.[41] The more motor units that are activated, the more muscle fibers are stimulated and the greater the muscle contraction. Lifting a heavy weight recruits more motor units and creates a more forceful muscle contraction than lifting a lighter weight.

Studies show that motor units come in different sizes and that smaller motor units are recruited first, followed by larger motor units. This rule is often referred to as the **size principle**.[52] Small motor units are recruited first because the impulse needed to activate them is less than that needed by larger motor units.[52] Another way of saying this is that smaller motor units stimulate slow-twitch, type I fibers while larger motor units stimulate fast-twitch, type II fibers. It is because of the size principle that type I fibers are recruited first, followed by type IIa and then type IIb. This actually makes sense in practical circumstances. For example, if you were carrying this book to your car, you would want to use only your type I fibers. If you instead used your type IIb fibers, they might fatigue before you reached your car, causing you to drop the book.

Delayed Onset Muscle Soreness

The feeling of pain or discomfort in muscles on days following a strenuous or unaccustomed activity is called **delayed onset muscle soreness** (DOMS). Any activity that is intense enough or to which the body is not accustomed will cause DOMS if you perform it for a long enough period of time. Such activities could include anything from shoveling snow to going out and running around the block one time. The pain usually occurs 24–72 hours following exercise and usually subsides within 7–10 days of the soreness-initiating event. Muscles during this time are said to be stiff, and there is often a decreased range of motion. During this time, people report a reduced ability to produce force in the affected muscles. Thus, people may not be able to lift as much weight when they experience DOMS. Research has shown that this is the result of both a decreased ability of the muscle to produce force and an unwillingness on the part of the person to use the DOMS-affected muscles.[115] Interestingly, DOMS is not felt when the muscle is at rest; rather, we only feel the pain when the muscles in question are moved or when the muscles are touched.[116] This fact can sometimes help fitness trainers to differentiate between DOMS and some other more serious types of pain (e.g., tendonitis). In other words, an absence of pain when not moving may be a clue that the person is experiencing DOMS.

DOMS does not result in any long-term damage to muscles. However, there is evidence of short-term damage. Muscle biopsies during DOMS reveal damage to key areas of muscle structure.[117] For example, studies show physical damage to sarcomeres as well as to their associated connective tissues. They also reveal elevations in various enzymes associated with tissue injury.

There are several theories to explain why DOMS occurs. All theories have merit, but no theory fully explains the process. The most common theories are the **torn tissue theory**, **connective tissue theory**, and **inflammation theory**.

Theories of DOMS

Theory	Main Details
Torn Tissue Theory	Damage to muscles is the cause of DOMS
Connective Tissue Theory	Damage to connective tissue is the cause of DOMS
Inflammation Theory	White blood cells release chemicals that sensitize pain receptors

These theories aside, what everyone agrees upon is that eccentric activities (e.g., walking downhill or lowering a dumbbell), also called "negatives," result in far more DOMS than concentric movements.[119]

Some may take various drugs like aspirin or other non-steroidal anti-inflammatory drugs (NSAIDs) to alleviate DOMS. While this practice helps reduce pain, it may not be the best practice for elite athletes. There is evidence that NSAIDs reduce protein synthesis following eccentric exercise.[120] This, in theory, might prolong DOMS and reduce athletic performance. For most people, however, this effect is probably not significant.

One common misconception involves lactic acid. There is no proof that lactic acid causes DOMS. Also, as stated previously, the body does not make lactic acid. People who say this likely confuse muscle burning during exercise with muscle pain (DOMS) the next day, but these are not the same thing.

Another common misconception about DOMS involves stretching. To date, there is not much evidence that stretching sore muscles alleviates DOMS. In fact, some evidence suggests that stretching can actually cause DOMS if a person is unaccustomed to stretching.[118] Stretching between sets, however, may speed recovery during subsequent sets. Likewise, the impact of various nutritional supplements (e.g., antioxidants) to protect against DOMS or to speed relief has, at best, mixed results and is not fully accepted.[38] As for so-called sports creams, these mask pain with either sensations of heat or cold without actually speeding recovery from DOMS. Currently, the only accepted therapy for reducing DOMS is performing a submaximal bout of exercise before the actual workout.[122] In other words, do one set of an exercise a day or so before doing 3 sets. In practical terms, novices who perform one set and gradually build upon this over time are less likely to experience DOMS or more serious injuries than those who partake in more aggressive exercise routines. For more information about this topic, see my review, "The Mystery of DOMS," which you may find at Joe-Cannon.com.

Types of Muscle Fibers

There are basically three types of muscle tissue in the body: smooth muscle (in blood vessels), cardiac muscle (in the heart), and skeletal muscle (biceps, triceps, etc.). This section deals only with skeletal muscle.

Skeletal muscle is called "skeletal" because, for the most part, it is attached to the skeleton. Skeletal muscle is also called voluntary muscle because we voluntarily cause it to move. For example, the biceps muscle cannot automatically lift a dumbbell—we must first think, "Lift that dumbbell," before our muscle can perform the action.

Skeletal muscle can be further divided into **type I muscle fibers** and **type II muscle fibers**, including various subtypes of each. The type I and type II fibers are also sometimes called slow-twitch and fast-twitch muscle fibers, respectively, where the "twitch" refers to contraction speed. In other words, slow-twitch fibers twitch or contract more slowly than fast-twitch fibers. Type II fibers can be further subdivided into different subtypes. Usually, we discuss **type IIa fibers** and **type IIb fibers.** Let us examine each in more detail now.

Type I muscle fibers are small fibers that produce low amounts of force. Because they can produce force for long periods of time, type I fibers are hard to fatigue. This is because they are aerobic fibers that contain an abundance of myoglobin (an oxygen-carrying molecule similar to hemoglobin), mitochondria, and capillaries, which allow them to burn fat and glucose for energy. They are purely aerobic fibers and generally do not have the ability to work anaerobically. Type I fibers do not show as much hypotrophy as other fiber types and are used during activities that are not very strenuous. They are called type I because they are usually the first muscle fibers activated when a muscle contracts. They are also called slow-twitch fibers because they contract more slowly than fast-twitch fibers (about 110 milliseconds vs. about 50 milliseconds for type II fibers). Another term for type I fibers sometimes used in academic settings is **slow oxidative fibers**. This term is more descriptive, referring to both the fibers' slow twitch properties as well as their ability to oxidize (i.e., burn) fat and sugar aerobically. Type I fibers used to be called "red fibers" because they are rich in mitochondria, which contain red-colored pigments called cytochromes.

Type IIa muscle fibers are "middle-of-the-road" fibers. They are not only larger than type I fibers and smaller than type IIb fibers, but they also generate much more force than type I fibers. Moreover, they also are able to sustain the force produced for longer periods of time. These fibers are used during a variety of activities such as resistance training, hiking, and sprinting. Thus, type II muscle fibers are both aerobic and anaerobic. While sometimes called fast twitch, another term used is **fast oxidative glycolytic** (FOG). This term refers to their ability to burn fat and sugar aerobically and anaerobically. They also utilize the creatine energy system.

Type IIb fibers are the most powerful fibers in the body. They contract the most quickly of all known fiber types, but the power that they produce does not last long. Thus, type IIb fibers are also the quickest to fatigue and have low endurance.[52] The reason for this is that they have the lowest number of mitochondria and capillaries (both of which are needed to burn fat). Type IIb fibers are strictly anaerobic fibers and basically use glucose (and creatine) to generate force. Because they are fast-twitch and rely upon glycolysis and other anaerobic means to generate force, they are sometimes called **fast glycolytic fibers** (FG). These fibers have the thickest diameter and are used during activities that are perceived to be very demanding such as powerlifting, bodybuilding (depending on the load lifted), and sprinting. It is important to note that fitness level dictates what is easy versus what is difficult. For some people, getting out of a chair is very difficult! Interestingly, research shows that, with exercise training, type IIb fibers begin to develop characteristics of type IIa fibers.[62,77] This may be the body's way of adapting to exercise. In other words, type IIa fibers are more useful than type IIb in that they are almost as powerful and can do a lot of things that type IIb cannot.

Quick Reference

Muscle Fiber Type	Brief Description
Smooth muscle	Lines blood vessels.
Cardiac muscle	Heart muscle. Also called involuntary muscle because it can contract on its own.
Skeletal muscle	Mostly attached to skeleton. Also called voluntary muscle.
Type I muscle fibers	Aerobic fibers. Endurance fibers. Burn fat and glucose.
Type IIa muscle fibers	Both aerobic & anaerobic. Strength & endurance fibers.
Type IIb muscle fibers	Totally anaerobic. Power fibers. Fatigue very fast.

People may have had problems naming muscle fibers in the past because different books may use different terms. The following table sorts through the confusion.

Muscle Fibers Types: Old Names and New Names

Commonly-used name	Commonly-used name	Older name	Technical name
Type I fibers	Slow twitch	Red fibers	Slow oxidative fibers (SO fibers)
Type IIa fibers	Fast twitch	Pink fibers	Fast oxidative glycolytic fibers (FOG fibers)
Type IIb fibers	Fast twitch	White fibers	Fast glycolytic fibers (FG fibers)

How Many Muscle Fiber Types Do We Have?

It appears that humans possess many different subtypes of muscle fibers besides type I and type II, which are normally discussed. Thus, some may read about other fiber types, including type IIAB, type IIx, and type IIc. These other types can be thought of as hybrids of the major types. In fitness, however, we usually only discuss type I, IIa, and IIb fibers.

How Many Type I and Type II Fibers Do We Have?

It is sometimes stated that adults have roughly 50% slow twitch and 50% fast twitch fibers. The problem with this statement, though, is that it is practically impossible to prove. Intuitively, it makes sense that people are blessed with both endurance as well as strength and power fibers. However, the only way to really confirm this is to take a biopsy of muscle. Since there are over 600 muscles in the body, this is not ethically or practically possible to do. What we can say is that different muscles tend to have different percentages of type I and type II fibers. For example, the abdominals tend to have high concentrations of slow twitch, type I fibers, while the leg muscles tend to have higher concentrations of fast twitch, type II fibers. Also, some research indicates that some endurance athletes have greater concentrations of type I fibers, while strength and power athletes may have more type II fibers.[53] Thus, genetics plays a role in fiber distribution. Other research of biopsied muscle has noted that young men tend to have more type IIa fibers in their vastus lateralis, while women tend to have more type I fibers.[54] The bottom line is that people have both type I and type II fibers, but the amount each can vary among people and is open to speculation.

Some have tried to devise ways of estimating muscle fiber type dominance by way of exercise.[55, 56] One method of doing so is based on first determining 1RM and then performing as many repetitions as possible using 80% of 1RM.[57] If the person can perform more than 12 repetitions, then that muscle group is said to be composed of at least 50% type I fibers. If they can do fewer than 7 repetitions, then the muscle group is at least 50% type IIb fibers. If they perform between 7–12 repetitions, then the muscle group supposedly has equal percentages of type I and type II fibers. "Recipes" like this and others are sometimes cited on websites, but they have not been clinically well studied. Another option is to look at the sports at which the person excels. Theoretically, excelling at aerobic sports might indicate more type I fibers, while experiencing success in anaerobic activities might mean that the athlete has more type II fibers. Again, without good science, this is merely speculation.

Do Men Have More Muscle Fibers Than Women?

Generally speaking, men tend to be stronger than women because they have a greater overall amount of muscle than women. However, a type I or type II muscle fiber from a woman is the same as that of a man and responds the same to exercise training.[62,76] It also appears that men and women have relatively similar percentages of type I and type II fibers per muscle group.[76] Women do tend to be weaker in upper body strength relative to men, but this has more to do with men having greater upper body muscle density than with their fibers being stronger.[76] Because of the fiber type resemblance between genders, it is generally not necessary to train women differently than men.

Can Women Develop Large Muscles?

The fear of developing large, manly muscles has unfortunately discouraged some women from lifting weights. However, this will not happen for the vast majority of women, because most do not have enough anabolic hormones (e.g., testosterone) to facilitate drastic muscle growth. While there are very muscular women in the world (such as female bodybuilders), they must usually train for many years, lifting very heavy weights, to become that bulky. These women also eat many more calories and a greater amount of protein than most. Others may also have genetic advantages such as naturally higher levels of testosterone or higher percentages of type II muscle fibers. Still others may use anabolic steroids. Sometimes, overweight women describe how they "get big" from strength training, but this may be due to their slightly enlarged muscles expanding the overlapping adipose tissue (fat), giving the impression that their muscles have grown greatly in size. Reducing calorie intake and adding some aerobic exercise should help reduce adipose girth. While it is possible that the muscles of some women may exhibit hypertrophy, this is outside of the norm and generally does not occur.

Can Exercise Alter Muscle Fiber Type?

Can exercise change type I fibers into type II fibers or vice versa? If a change of this nature is possible, it is more likely that what actually occurs are alterations in the chemical composition of fiber types rather than one fiber transforming into another. For example, aerobic training might increase the aerobic capacity of type IIa fibers, while anaerobic training might decrease the aerobic capacity. Currently, there is no real proof that exercise training can physically change a type I fiber into a type II fiber.[62]

People who are usually interested in this question are athletes. However, athletic performance is not simply about fiber type. Practice and determination are also involved. As evidence of this, remember that one of the greatest athletes of all time, Michael Jordan, was once cut from his high school basketball team.

Can We Make More Muscle Cells?

The technical term for making new cells is "hyperplasia." While the primary process whereby muscles grow in size and strength is through hypertrophy, there is evidence that, under some extreme conditions, we may be able to make more muscle cells. Most of the support for hyperplasia stems from animals subjected to long periods of stress.[59] With respect to humans, some controversial research of highly trained bodybuilders finds larger muscles (i.e., triceps) than in non-bodybuilders, while the size of individual muscle fibers between the two groups was not different.[60] This hints that hyperplasia may occur under some stressful exercise conditions. Not all studies, though, agree with this finding.[61] Other evidence for hyperplasia includes **satellite cells** (undifferentiated proto-muscle cells) and **muscle fiber splitting** (where one muscle cell splits into two). What can be said for now is that, if hyperplasia of muscle cells occurs, the process of how to make it happen is open to speculation. Moreover, because it has not been directly observed in humans, its impact on muscle size and strength may not be significant. If it does occur, it may be limited only to those involved in very intense exercise over a prolonged period of time.

Atrophy

Muscle atrophy refers to a reduction in muscle size and strength. In most people, atrophy begins after about three weeks of not working out. For highly trained athletes, on the other hand, it may occur even sooner.[41] During this process, muscle proteins begin to break down faster than the rate of protein synthesis. Eventually, this results in a loss of muscle strength and size. This lack of strength, coupled with an increase in connective tissue between muscle fibers makes it difficult for people to perform activities of daily living (ADLs) and increases stiffness. Over time, this may result in depression, loss of productivity, and, if taken to its ultimate conclusion, confinement to a nursing home. Exercise—especially weight-bearing resistance training—is one of the best ways to combat muscle atrophy. When prescribing activities to reduce atrophy, fitness professionals should consider the limitations of the client and, if possible, design activities that overload weakened muscles just a little more than they are used. Activities that resemble ADLs can also be great help in improving this condition.

Besides less frequent exercise, atrophy can also result from poor nutrition, inadequate calories and protein, eating disorders, lack of anabolic hormones (e.g., testosterone or GH), reduced nervous stimulation to an area, and even too much bed rest, to name a few. In addition, various diseases (cancer, COPD, and others) may result in muscle atrophy. Because so many conditions can lead to this condition, the fitness professional should consider this when evaluating his or her clients.

Conditions Where Atrophy May Be Observed*

Inactivity	Sedentary jobs	Anorexia Nervosa	Poor nutrition
Cancer	HIV/AIDS	Bulimia	Inadequate protein
COPD	Prolonged bed rest	Burns	Depression
Immobilization	Parkinson's disease	Stroke	Aging process
Arthritis	Prednisone therapy	Injury	Diabetes

*Not a complete list

Sarcopenia

In general, people gain strength up to the age of 30, after which it slowly begins to decline.[66] First coined in 1989, the term **sarcopenia** refers to a type of atrophy associated with age-related loss of muscle size and strength.[63] After age 30, people tend to lose 0.5 % of muscle mass per year until the age of 50.[66] After 50, the loss of muscle accelerates.[65] While all muscle fibers are affected by sarcopenia, the condition targets type II muscle fibers the most.[67,69] This probably is at least partially related to the reduced use of these fibers as people age. The loss of type II fibers has profound implications for loss of mobility and independence as we grow older. As such, fitness professionals should have an understanding of this process so that they can not only recognize the signs of sarcopenia, but so that they may help people cope with it more effectively as well.

It is important to distinguish between sarcopenia and other similar conditions such as **muscle wasting** and **cachexia**. Muscle wasting refers to muscle loss resulting from lack of use or from disease. It can occur at any age and is usually referred to as "atrophy." In adults, a BMI of less than 18.5 sometimes indicates muscle wasting. Cachexia, on the other hand, is more frequently associated with diseases such as cancer. Sarcopenia is different from these in that it is specifically related to the aging process.

Atrophy Conditions: How They Differ

Muscle wasting	Atrophy stemming from disuse
Cachexia	Disease-induced muscle and weight loss
Sarcopenia	Age-related muscle loss

Both men and women develop sarcopenia; however, some research suggests that men (possibly because of their greater muscle mass) may experience sarcopenia to a greater degree than women.[63] For example, some research has noted that 58% of men over the age of 75 had sarcopenia, compared to 45% of women of the same age. However, because women tend to live longer, they may be at greater risk of experiencing the ravages of sarcopenia for longer periods of time. Currently, the reason why sarcopenia occurs is unknown, and there are likely many factors that lead to this condition. One factor over which we have no control is genetics. Additionally, sarcopenia may be part of the aging process and may be affected by reductions in anabolic hormones. Muscle fiber stimulation from the nervous system appears to decrease as we get older because of a gradual loss of motor units, and muscle cells that are no longer stimulated die off. As we age, we may also be less efficient at making muscle proteins.[70] This condition is called **anabolic resistance.** Some research finds a 30% reduction in muscle protein synthesis as we age.[65] Levels of myostatin, a protein that reduces muscle growth, may also rise with age.[71] As an aside, some supplements are touted to naturally block the effects of myostatin, promising muscle growth without any effort. Fitness professionals should remember that many of these supplements lack proper research.[72] For a better understanding of "myostatin blockers," read my book, *Nutritional Supplements: What Works and Why*, available at www.Joe-Cannon.com. Regardless of myostatin's effects, evidence does suggest that resistance training can stimulate protein synthesis in older men and women.[73]

Unlike genetics, the choices that we make about how we live also play a critical role in the development of sarcopenia. For example, lack of physical exercise probably accelerates sarcopenia. As people age, they are generally less likely to engage in resistance training, which helps preserve type II fibers. Moreover, aging individuals may avoid tasks that they deem too difficult to perform, such as weight lifting or carrying groceries. Many older individuals continue to walk as they get older, but walking mostly enlists endurance-oriented type I fibers. The lack of appropriate stimulation of type II fibers (especially through eccentric actions associated with strength training) as we age is probably one of the main reasons for their selective decline with sarcopenia.

Poor nutrition can also impact sarcopenia. People tend to eat fewer calories and protein as they grow older. In the absence of adequate calories and protein, the body, in an attempt to stay alive, can cannibalize itself to obtain the energy that it needs. Gluconeogenesis refers to the creation of glucose from non-carbohydrate energy sources such as protein. In essence, the body may begin to degrade its own protein, turn it into sugar, and burn it for energy. In the absence of proper amounts of exercise, the body may choose to degrade muscle fibers that are no longer being used (type II fibers). This may be one of the reasons why type II fibers are decimated in sarcopenia. As type II fibers dwindle, it becomes even more difficult to perform ADLs. When a person does move, they do so more slowly, which in turn may increase their risk of injury. For example, those with sarcopenia may take longer to cross the street if a traffic light suddenly changes or may be less likely to catch themselves if they fall. Fitness professionals should remember that, in some older people, the sensation of thirst also may decrease, leading to reduced fluid consumption, dehydration, and fatigue. This in turn, may result in even less activity, further advancing sarcopenia.

The loss of strength accompanying sarcopenia may lead to less aerobic activity (e.g., walking), which can contribute to elevations in cholesterol, LDL, and triglycerides with corresponding decreases in HDL. Ultimately, this promotes the development of or exacerbates the severity of heart disease. The loss of muscle may also contribute to type II diabetes. Muscle burns calories, and the loss of muscle accompanying sarcopenia leaves less muscle available to use the calories consumed during a meal. In theory, this means that higher insulin levels are needed to store the extra calories as fat. Chronically high insulin levels might reduce the number of insulin receptors, leading to insulin resistance, metabolic syndrome, and ultimately type II diabetes.[67,68] Diabetes further escalates the risk of a number of complications related to heart disease.

Because muscle is involved with metabolic rate (the speed at which we burn calories), sarcopenia can lead to a lower BMR. Some have estimated that from age 30–80, there is approximately a 15% decrease in BMR.[65] This can lead to weight gain, making people even slower and less likely to exercise.

Sometimes fitness trainers can recognize sarcopenia by looking at the lower body. Remember that the thighs and buttocks usually have a high percentage of type II fibers. People whose thighs and buttocks are thinner or smaller in comparison to the rest of the body may have this condition. At the other end of the spectrum are those who are very overweight. Because being overweight or obese limits activity, sarcopenia may develop in these cases as well. This condition is called **obesity-related sarcopenia.**

Sarcopenia is a term not often mentioned in fitness circles. Regardless, it is safe to say that every person reading these words will be impacted by this condition eventually. Considering that America is quickly becoming a nation of older people, the ravages of sarcopenia have profound implications for not only the health care system, but, in this author's opinion, national security as well. By recognizing sarcopenia, fitness professionals—more than any other health care specialist—have a unique opportunity to be at the forefront of the public's education of this often overlooked phenomenon.

Sarcopenia May Contribute To

Increased incidence of falls	Reduced ability to perform ADLs	Poor quality of life
Reduced strength	Lack of independence	Depression
Slower speed	Confinement to a nursing home	Compromised immune system
Lower aerobic capacity	Reduced metabolic rate	Early death

Types of Muscle Actions

Essentially, there are three different types of muscle actions (muscle contractions) usually discussed. They are **isometric** muscle actions, **isokinetic** muscle actions and **isotonic** (dynamic) muscle actions. Of these types, isometric and isotonic actions are what fitness trainers most frequently encounter. Let us now discuss each type in greater detail.

Isometric Muscle Actions

The prefix "iso" means "same," while "metric" means "distance," so isometric muscle actions occur when no change in muscle length occurs as the muscle is used. There is also no change in joint angle during isometric muscle actions. Other names referring to isometrics include **static contractions** and **dynamic muscle tension**. An example of this type of muscle action is the plank exercise. Pressing the hands together in front of the chest as hard as possible is another example. The core muscles of the trunk also isometrically contract during everyday activities. Isometric muscle actions were popular in the early 20th century but eventually fell out of favor with strength trainers and were replaced with more popular isotonic muscle actions. Some weightlifters still incorporate them into their exercise routines through practices such as holding the contraction for a second or two at the end of each repetition. Isometrics by themselves increase muscle strength, but they are less effective than isotonic muscle actions. The reason for this is that the joint angle is fixed in isometric exercises. For example, pressing the hands together in front of the chest as hard as possible may increase strength, but if an object was then placed between the hands to adjust the joint angle, force production would decrease. In other words, by not moving the muscle through its full safe range of motion, strength development over that ROM is compromised. Conflicting evidence also suggests that isometric exercise may either increase or reduce blood pressure. As such, people with uncontrolled hypertension may want to avoid this type of activity.[47]

Isokinetic Muscle Actions

The prefix "iso" means "same" and "kinetic" refers to speed or movement. Thus, isokinetic muscle actions are those that occur at the same speed throughout the range of motion. When we exercise, our muscles typically do not move at a fixed rate of speed, so this type of muscle action does not mimic what we do in real life. Performing isokinetic movements requires the use of equipment such as what may be seen in physical therapy. Indeed, physical therapists may use isokinetic exercises that only allow the muscle to move at a specific speed. The advantage of this type of muscle action is that the muscle can exert maximum force throughout the ROM. Some health clubs may have a piece of equipment called an **upper body ergometer** (UBE) in which the person rotates his or her arms in a circular fashion. One of the settings on the UBE is an isokinetic mode in which you can set the machine to only move at a certain speed. Nothing can make the machine to move faster than the speed to which it is set. As an aside, the UBE can also be of help during shoulder rehab or can provide an aerobic workout to those who are in wheelchairs.

Isotonic Muscle Actions

This is the type of muscle action that we engage most frequently. The term "isotonic" refers to constant tension being produced inside the muscle and how the muscle length changes as we go through a movement's safe range of motion (ROM). Isotonic muscle actions are composed of two phases—**concentric** and **eccentric**. If we limit the discussion to strength training, concentric muscle actions (sometimes called **positives**) occur when we are lifting the weight. If we could look at the muscle cell during a concentric muscle action, we would see that the actin and myosin proteins slide closer together to shorten muscle length. Eccentric muscle actions (sometimes called **negatives**) usually occur when we are lowering a weight. During eccentric actions, we would observe the actin and myosin proteins in the muscle being pulled apart. Thus, during eccentric muscle actions, the muscle lengthens as force is applied to it.

Eccentric muscle actions can result in greater improvements of strength and higher metabolic rates than concentric movements. The downside is that eccentrics also result in more frequent delayed onset muscle soreness (DOMS).[48] Sometimes people call eccentric exercises "eccentric muscle contractions." However, this is technically a misnomer since a muscle cannot contract when it is elongating. This is why you see the term "eccentric muscle actions" used more often.

Types of Muscle Actions: How They Compare

	Isometric	Isokinetic	Isotonic
Joint movement	None	Yes	Yes
Speed of movement	None	Constant	Varies
Force generation	Constant	Variable	Constant
Change in fiber length	No	Yes	Yes

Do Muscles Have a Memory?

The concept of "muscle memory" refers to the phenomenon whereby trained muscles, after a period of non-use (e.g., not working out for a few months), appear to regain their strength at a faster rate than they originally did when training first began. In reality, what is referred to as muscle memory is probably better described as "brain-muscle memory" because the brain relays instructions muscles to perform a movement. In some circles, this type of memory is referred to as **procedural memory** because the brain is remembering how to perform a procedure. For example, we have all heard the phrase, "You never forget how to ride a bike." No matter how long it has been since you rode a bicycle, you pick the skill up faster than when you first learned it. With respect to exercise, one study has noted that sedentary women who strength trained for 20 weeks, stopped for 30–32 weeks, and then lifted again for 6 weeks regained strength more quickly than they did at the start of the study. [88] In addition, cross sectional area (i.e., thickness) of type II fibers also increased more rapidly than at the start of the study. The mechanisms behind muscle memory are not well understood, but probably involve the interaction of the brain and central nervous system with muscles.

Strength Training and Testosterone

Testosterone is primarily produced by the Leydig cells of the testes and, to a lesser degree, by the adrenal glands. While typically considered a male hormone, women also make testosterone in the ovaries and adrenal glands, albeit to a lesser degree than men. In men, testosterone levels are usually highest in the morning and lower over the course of the day.[78] Testosterone impacts a number of organ systems, with the muscles being the most notable. Following secretion, testosterone travels through the blood, usually attached to a specialized protein (sex hormone binding globulin or SHBG) that acts to inhibit the hormone's action.[90] Most of the circulating testosterone is bound to this or other proteins and is not thought to be active. In contrast, about 0.2–2% is the active, free testosterone.[90] At its target sites, testosterone binds to testosterone receptors on the cell's surface and, through a complex series of reactions within the cell's brain center (nucleus), impacts a myriad of functions ranging from muscle growth and repair to immune function support and libido, to name a few.

Strength training is a well-known contributor to increasing testosterone levels. Following a single bout of strength training, testosterone levels rise temporarily and then drop about an hour later.[90] Other research finds that testosterone increases after a single bout of aerobic exercise as well.[93] However, long term aerobic exercise (such as a marathon) appears to depress testosterone levels.[94]

The time for which testosterone levels remain depressed after resistance training is debatable and probably varies with a number of factors, including type of exercise, intensity, and volume. The degree of secretion also depends on several factors. For example, compound exercises (e.g., squats) elicit a greater surge in testosterone than do single joint exercises (e.g., biceps curls). It also appears that performing large-muscle exercises first elicits a greater response than performing exercises that use smaller muscle groups first. The resistance used also plays a role, with heavier resistances (i.e., 5RM–10 RM) resulting in a greater magnitude of release than lighter resistances. Likewise, performing multiple sets appears superior to completing single sets. The volume of exercise refers to the total amount of weight lifted and is found by multiplying sets by number of repetitions by amount of resistance used. It appears that testosterone levels elevate more with moderate to high volumes of exercise. According to some research, at least 4 sets might be needed to elevate testosterone, although in less fit individuals, fewer sets may do just as well.[91]

Exercise Factors Involved in Raising Testosterone Levels

Large muscle exercises	Volume: high to moderate
Heavy resistance (85–95% 1RM)	Rest: 30 sec to 1 min between sets

There is also some evidence that experienced lifters (> 2 years) may see greater testosterone surges than novice lifters.[92] This may be at least partially due to experienced lifters' abilities to engage in the intense training thought required to elicit testosterone elevations.

Alcohol consumption is one factor that has not received a lot of attention in terms of exercise. However, a review of the evidence suggests that it can reduce free and bound testosterone in both men and women.[90] In theory, this might upset the testosterone to estrogen ratio and impact muscle and strength development. Based on some evidence, consuming more than 12 ounces of beer can reduce testosterone levels in men, while up to 12 ounces might temporarily raise testosterone levels.[90]

Strength Training or Cardio First?

Some trainers may advocate that strength training should be performed before cardio if both activities are included in the same workout. Is this always the best advice? One small study noted that the answer may not be as clear as once believed. In this study, a small group of men either lifted first or did cardio first. The researchers noted that, while total testosterone levels after performing strength training first were indeed higher than when cardio was performed first, the levels dropped rather quickly. On the other hand, when cardio was performed before strength training, testosterone levels continued to rise and remained higher at the end of the measuring period. So, what is better for muscle development? More research is needed, but the bigger question that personal trainers must ask is what is in the best interest of the client? For most clients—especially in the beginning—exercising is not about getting bigger or stronger, but about being healthy. Obviously, the exercise prescription should be based on the needs and abilities of the client rather than on urban legends or research studies using people who may or may not reflect your typical client.

Supplements and Testosterone

Can dietary supplements raise testosterone levels? This author is skeptical of most products because of their lack of published, peer reviewed research. Most dietary supplements have no such evidence and instead rely on research related to their individual ingredients (e.g., tribulus or fenugreek). Moreover, the evidence for many popular ingredients is also less than spectacular. Personal trainers should always ask for published, peer reviewed studies of humans when deciding whether or not a supplement works. For information on many reputed testosterone boosters, as well as other products, see the reviews at SupplementClarity.com.

Strength Training and Growth Hormone

Human growth hormone (GH or HGH), also called somatotropin, is a protein-based hormone secreted from the anterior pituitary gland that acts to strengthen tendons, bones, as well as muscles. GH also plays other roles, including immune system support. While generally considered a single hormone, GH actually represents a family of related compounds. With respect to resistance training, GH stimulates the use of amino acids, which contributes to protein synthesis and muscle hypertrophy, while at the same time decreasing protein breakdown and speeding up tissue repair. Other effects of GH include decreased use of glucose for fuel and increased fat usage.

Effects of Growth Hormone

Enhances fat breakdown (lipolysis)	Promotes gluconeogenesis	Possible bone growth stimulation[*]
Stimulates immune system	Promotes protein anabolism	Possible increased epidermis thickness[*]
Stimulates cartilage growth	Decreases glycogen synthesis	Possible increase in LBM[*]

* see reference 96

With respect to strength training, multiple sets incorporating exercises that recruit large muscle groups coupled with heavy loads (e.g., 10 RM) and short rest periods (30–60 seconds) appear to be best for significantly elevating GH release.[95] Notice that protocols to elevate GH are similar to those required to elevate testosterone. GH levels may remain elevated for 15–30 minutes postexercise.[95]

Many of the effects attributed to GH are actually the result of other compounds called **insulin-like growth factors** (IGFs), which are secreted by the liver when stimulated by GH. They are called "IGFs" because they resemble the hormone insulin. The term **somatomedin** is another name for IGFs. It is important to note that there are several members of the IGF family of compounds.

Sometimes GH is touted as the "fountain of youth." Most claims on this issue stem from a 1990 study of 6 months of GH injections in older men.[96] This study found that in older men (with low GH levels), GH injections resulted in reduced body fat (14.4%), increased lumbar vertebrae thickness (1.6%), and increased skin thickness (7.1%). However, this study involved GH injections, which are very different than orally taken products. Many GH-boosting supplements contain the amino acids arginine and ornithine. While large doses of these amino acids may slightly elevate GH in some people, they have never been shown to boost strength or muscle hypertrophy.[38] Side effects from GH injections include but may not be limited to unhealthy growth of the heart (cardiomyopathy), carpal tunnel syndrome, insulin resistance (which can increase diabetes risk), and unhealthy enlargement of the kidneys and bones.[95]

Growth Hormone: Possible Side Effects

Joint pain	Cardiomyopathy	Increase lean body mass
Carpal tunnel syndrome	Fluid retention	Decreased fat mass
Insulin resistance	Possible increased cancer risk	Elevated blood pressure[*]

* see reference 96

Cortisol

Cortisol is also called adrenocortical steroid because it is made in the adrenal glands (located on top of the kidneys) after being stimulated by the hypothalamus gland of the brain. While testosterone is considered an anabolic hormone, cortisol is probably what most fitness people think of when they hear the word "catabolic." One reason for this is that the hormone facilitates gluconeogenesis, the conversion of amino acids and other compounds into glucose. It also inhibits protein synthesis, serving to increase blood sugar levels during times of fasting. In this respect, cortisol acts similarly to glucagon, which also raises blood sugar levels.

Like testosterone, most cortisol in the blood is thought to be bound by proteins (called corticosteroid-binding globulin) as it travels through the body. Only about 10% of the hormone is the free, "active" form. Normally, cortisol levels rise quickly in response to a stressor, whether it is low blood sugar, surgery, or intense exercise. With respect to exercise, avoiding cortisol does not seem to be an option. Studies show that the same types of activities that elicit testosterone and GH release also result in cortisol increases. The good news, however, is that regular exercise appears to reduce the effects of cortisol.[77] This appears to be true in both untrained and exercise-trained individuals.[111] Extremely intense exercise training, however, in the absence of adequate rest and nutrition, may increase cortisol, resulting in the development of **overtraining syndrome.** High-volume, high-intensity exercise, coupled with short rest periods, appears to augment cortisol more than lower intensity routines. The rest period between sets also appears to impact cortisol levels, with longer rest periods (3 minutes) promoting a lower amount released than that observed along with shorter rest periods (1 minute).[102] Ironically, this protocol describes many popular **high intensity training** (HIT) programs. However, adequate rest, sound nutrition, and proper exercise program design can help reduce any possible deleterious effects of this hormone. As mentioned previously, cortisol is involved with the degradation of muscle tissue. Some research finds that fast-twitch, type II fibers are more affected by cortisol than slow-twitch, type I fibers.[77]

While traditionally thought of as a "bad" hormone, cortisol is intimately involved in the development of strength and plays a critical role in rebuilding muscle after exercise has occurred. Exercise is a stressor and does cause damage to muscle—it is the repair process that causes muscle to grow in strength. By taking part in the rebuilding process, cortisol helps muscles adapt over time.

Rhabdomyolysis

Rhabdomyolysis (rhab-doe-my-oh-lie-sis) basically means "muscle fiber death" and is a very serious disorder in which muscle cells rupture from a stress that is applied too quickly for the body to adapt. This overwhelms the body, causing muscle fibers to die. When exercise is the stressor, this is called **exertional** or **exercise-induced rhabdomyolysis.** Because of the prevalence of high-intensity exercise programs, all fitness trainers need to be familiar with this condition and its symptoms.

As skeletal muscles rupture (die), they release their cellular contents into the blood, which can cause serious side effects. For example, the calcium and potassium released from muscles can, in extreme cases, cause a heart attack. Muscle cell hemoglobin, called myoglobin, is toxic to the kidneys and can cause kidney failure. People with rhabdomyolysis often require kidney dialysis for a period of time afterwards because of this. It is possible to die from rhabdomyolysis.[184] Exercise in hot environments as well as activities focusing on eccentric muscle actions also appear to increase its incidence. "Rhabdo," as it's often called, can occur after a single workout.[153] Trainers should remember that it is the quick increase in exercise intensity that often results in this condition. That said, what is too much for one person may not be too much in another, as is highlighted in a case report describing the occurrence of rhabdo in a 29-year-old man who reported performing only 30 sit-ups a day for 5 days.[155] This leaves open the possibility that some people may be more susceptible to rhabdo than others. Indeed, some genetic conditions (e.g., sickle cell anemia trait) do appear to increase the risk.[154] Rhabdo might also be increased in people who take cholesterol-lowering medications as well as some supplements. Cases of exertional rhabdomyolysis have been reported in the military, as well as in firemen, law enforcement trainees, football players, bodybuilders, and marathoners.[152,182] Case reports have also documented rhabdomyolysis arising as a result of overzealous personal trainers who push clients too hard.[153]

While medical tests can rapidly diagnosis this condition, fitness professionals may overlook it or mistake it for DOMS. They are not the same. For one thing, the pain from rhabdo often arises more quickly that the discomfort associated with DOMS.[152] People may report feeling sore almost immediately after halting exercise and up to 24 hours later. Also, unlike DOMS, rhabdo hurts when people are not moving. There may also be visual swelling of the muscles that might reduce range of motion. One possible visual sign of rhabdo is the presence of dark-colored (think reddish, ice tea color) urine, though this sign does not arise in every situation.[152] While dehydration during exercise can make rhabdo worse, it is important to remember that staying hydrated during exercise will not prevent rhabdo from occurring.

Rhabdo is often discussed within the context of high-intensity or extreme exercise programs. However, fitness trainers must remember that *any* type of exertion used while training a more susceptible person can cause this condition. Since it is not possible to look at someone and determine their risk, trainers should refrain from intense, bodybuilding-type, multiple-set programs in beginners. Doing so increases the risk of not only causing rhabdo, but of being sued because of an incident as well. This author believes that all trainers who conduct boot camp-type workouts should educate members about the possibility of rhabdo.

For much more information about this condition, see my post, "Rhabdomyolysis and Personal Training: Facts You Need to Know," found at Joe-Cannon.com.

Rhabdomyolysis Signs and Symptoms

Intense muscle pain/weakness	Difficulty moving limbs	Reduced urination
Muscle pain when not moving	Feeling nauseous/vomiting	Fever
Visible muscle swelling	Confusion	Darkly colored urine

Chapter 7

CARDIOVASCULAR PHYSIOLOGY

The cardiovascular (CV) system is made up of a number of organs that assist with the transportation of oxygen, nutrients, and hormones as well as the removal of waste products. The main parts of the cardiovascular system are the heart, blood, and blood vessels. The lungs are also included because this is where the blood gives off its carbon dioxide and is infused with fresh oxygen.

The heart is the pump responsible for pushing blood through the CV system. The major blood vessels are called **arteries** and **veins.** A good way to remember each is to keep in mind that, in general, arteries carry oxygen-rich blood *away* from the heart, while veins return oxygen-depleted blood back to the heart. As blood travels further away from the heart, the arteries get increasingly smaller. Smaller arteries are called **arterioles**. These eventually get even smaller and are called **capillaries**. In capillaries, oxygen and other nutrients are exchanged for waste products. On the return trip back to the heart, small blood vessels called **venules** eventually widen into veins, which return blood to the heart.

Blood

The average human adult has about 10 pints of blood in his or her body. Blood is a tissue that consists of a watery portion, plasma, and a cellular portion. Just a few of the cells contained in blood are red blood cells (RBCs), while many are infection-fighting white blood cells (WBCs). The RBCs carry oxygen throughout the body. Specifically, every red blood cell can carry about 4 oxygen molecules.[22] Red blood cells are able to transport oxygen because they contain an iron-rich compound called **hemoglobin,** which is responsible for giving blood its red color. Red blood cells are made within bone marrow. An interesting fact about hemoglobin is that, as much as it likes oxygen, it *loves* carbon monoxide, an odorless yet toxic gas.[22] This is the reason why people may die if locked in the garage with the car running. Even in low concentrations, carbon monoxide can cause fatigue, chest pain, and impaired vision and coordination.[23] Cigarettes also contain carbon monoxide, which is one of the reasons why warning labels must mention its presence.

Functions of Blood*

• Carries oxygen	• Regulates temperature	• Remove waste products
• Blood clotting	• Regulates pH of blood	• Transports hormones

* Not a complete list

It is blood's ability to carry oxygen that is at the heart of many nutritional and pharmacological attempts to amplify blood volume. **Blood doping** is a generic term used to describe various ways to boost red blood cell production and enhance exercise performance. For example, one method involves injecting the hormone erythropoietin (EPO), which makes red blood cells. The body naturally produces EPO when it needs RBCs, but some athletes may also use it in the hopes that it will give them an advantage in their sport. Blood doping is illegal in many sports, including those in the Olympics, because it carries severe side effects, including death.[19] Increased red blood cell concentration means that the blood gets thicker (more viscous). During exercise, water loss increases the blood's viscosity even more. Eventually, the strain of pumping this gooey mess overwhelms the heart, which can result in a heart attack. One natural—and legal—way to enhance red blood cells is by exercising at higher altitudes. Greater altitudes have lower levels of breathable oxygen. After a few weeks, a body exercising in such an environment compensates by naturally making more red blood cells. It is important to remember, however, that exercise in general will increase red blood cell production no matter what the altitude is.

The Lungs

The lungs are crucial to the functioning of the cardiovascular system because they serve as the location where blood gives up the carbon dioxide (CO_2) that it picked up from working muscles and to be infused with fresh oxygen. Humans have two lungs—a left lung and a right lung. Far from just empty sacs in our chest, the lungs are very complex and have a surface area that, if stretched out, could cover more than a tennis court.[21] This fantastic surface area is integral to our ability to breathe and continue to live.

Air travels to the lungs via the **trachea.** Each lung is further subdivided into smaller airways called **bronchioles,** which eventually lead to small air sacs called **alveoli.** In the alveoli, the blood receives new oxygen and gives up carbon dioxide gas. Each of the 300 million alveoli that are present in the lungs are surrounded by tiny capillaries that allow for gas exchange to take place.[39] Gas exchange within the lungs is made possible by differing concentrations of oxygen and carbon dioxide. In simple terms, things move from where there is a lot of something to where there is less. Since there is more oxygen in the lungs than in the oxygen-depleted RBCs, oxygen enters the RBCs and bonds to hemoglobin. Since there is less CO_2 in the lungs than in the blood, CO_2 leaves the blood and is exhaled from the body. The reverse happens when oxygen-rich blood reaches the cells of your body, because the cells have a lot of CO_2 and little oxygen. The other reason why this happens is referred to as the **Bohr Effect.** This refers to the fact that the higher relative acidity of the working muscles weakens the chemical bond between hemoglobin and oxygen. A weaker bond means that oxygen is more likely to leave hemoglobin and go to the cells of the body, where it can be used to produce energy.

All humans have areas of the respiratory tract that do not take part in gas exchange. This is referred to as dead space. **Anatomic dead space** includes conducting pathways that do not take part in gas exchange, like the trachea and mouth. **Physiologic dead space,** on the other hand, refers to portions of the lungs that do not partake in gas exchange. Physiologic dead space takes up only small part of the lungs.

The control centers of breathing are found in the brain, specifically in a structure called the **medulla** (brain stem). The brain knows when to tell the lungs to inhale and exhale because it has specialized receptors called **chemoreceptors** that monitor the acidity of the blood. Because high levels of CO_2 indicate that the blood is becoming too acidic, when the brain detects that CO_2 levels are getting too high or too low, it sends a signal to the lungs to inhale. There are basically two different types of chemoreceptors: **central chemoreceptors** monitor CO_2 levels, and **peripheral chemoreceptors** keep tabs on oxygen levels. While both are important, the central chemoreceptors are most important because they keep track of CO_2 levels and also keep tabs on pH levels. Remember, the body does not want to be too acidic, as this can affect the overall physiological balance (**homeostasis**) of the body. Sometimes, when people go diving underwater, they first hyperventilate. When they do this, they breathe more quickly than they normally do. This lowers the CO_2 levels in the blood and resets the brain's signal to cause inhalation. In this way, divers are able to stay underwater for a little longer. Eventually though, the lack of oxygen is detected by the chemoreceptors and the body is required to breathe again.

With respect to the lungs, there are some terms with which to be familiar. They are:

1. **Tidal Volume:** The tidal volume is the volume of air that can be inhaled or exhaled in a single normal breath.[24] An average young adult inhales and exhales about a pint (500 mL) of air with each breath.[24]
2. **Vital Capacity:** The maximum volume of air that can be exhaled after the person has inhaled as much as they can.[24] In a young adult, this equals about a gallon of air (4600 mL).[24]
3. **Residual Volume.** Even after a person has exhaled as much as he or she can, some air will remain in the lungs. This is the residual volume. For an adult, this usually averages about 2 pints (1200 mL).[24]

These factors (especially the first two) are sometimes measured in athletes, so you may run into them one day if you train this population.

Basic Anatomy of the Heart

Of all muscles of the body, the heart is undoubtedly the most important. This organ, about the size of a fist, contracts an average of 100,000 times and pumps about 2,000 gallons of blood each day![18] For those who live until the age of 80, the heart performs at least 2.9 billion beats![41]

The human heart has four chambers: 2 **atria** and 2 **ventricles**. Between the atria and ventricles are a series of valves or flaps of connective tissue that make sure that blood only travels in one direction. The valve between the right atria and right ventricle is called the **tricuspid valve**. The valve between the left atria and left ventricle is called the **bicuspid** or **mitral valve**. The heart walls themselves are made up of three distinct layers: the outer **epicardium** layer, a middle layer called the **myocardium,** and an inner layer called the **endocardium.**

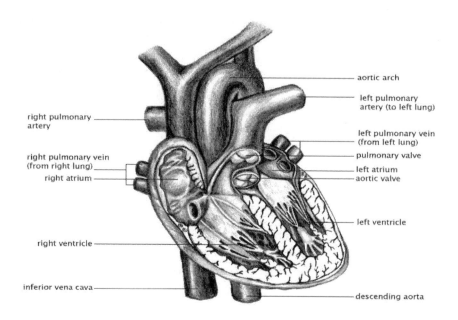

right pulmonary artery

right pulmonary vein (from right lung)

right atrium

right ventricle

inferior vena cava

aortic arch

left pulmonary artery (to left lung)

left pulmonary vein (from left lung)

pulmonary valve

left atrium

aortic valve

left ventricle

descending aorta

Heart Muscle Versus Skeletal Muscle

Both heart muscle and skeletal muscle are similar in that they are both striated, containing actin and myosin muscle proteins. They also both contract according to the sliding filament theory. They differ, however, in a few key areas. For one, heart muscle has the ability to contract on its own. This is ideal since nobody wants to keep remembering to tell their heart to beat! Another difference is that there is just one type of heart muscle, while there are different types of skeletal muscle (slow-twitch and fast-twitch). Specifically, heart muscle is very aerobic in nature, possessing many similarities to that of slow-twitch, type I fibers. Another important difference is that heart muscle cells are connected to each other by way of **intercalated disks**. The word "intercalate" means to insert between something. Intercalated disks are inserted between heart cells and allow for the speedy transmission of nerve impulses from one heart cell to another. It is because of intercalated disks that the heart is able to contract as a single unit.

The heart is furnished with its own blood supply via the **left** and **right coronary arteries,** which supply blood to the left and right sides of the heart, respectively. The coronary arteries begin as branching off points of the **aorta** and then further spread out over the heart to ensure adequate distribution of oxygen and nutrients throughout the myocardium. Blood leaves the heart by way of the coronary veins. For those who have trouble remembering which is which, remember that arteries contain high levels of oxygen and nutrients, while veins contain low levels.

The path that blood takes through the heart is as follows: Blood enters the heart via two large veins—the superior vena cava and inferior vena cava. Both of these veins empty into the right atrium of the heart. From the right atrium, blood travels to the right ventricle and passes into the lungs via the pulmonary arteries, where blood gives off its carbon dioxide and is infused with fresh oxygen. After this, blood leaves the lungs and passes into the left atrium and finally into the left ventricle. It is from the left ventricle that blood is ejected from the heart and travels to all parts of the body. Eventually, blood that is low in oxygen and nutrients returns to the heart again via the superior and inferior vena cava. This return of oxygen-poor blood to the heart is called **venous return.**

The heart muscle surrounding the left ventricle is thicker than that in other areas of the heart. This makes sense, as the force created by the contracting left ventricle is what propels the blood out of the heart. It is interesting to note that with exercise training, this left ventricular heart muscle actually gets stronger. A stronger left ventricle means that one can eject more blood out of the heart in a given moment of time. This is an example of one of the positive changes that occurs in the body when one engages in an exercise program.

When blood leaves the heart, it does so through its main artery—the aorta. As the aorta travels up the sides of the neck, it branches off and goes in different directions. The point at which the aorta branches off is subjected to high pressures as blood courses through the circulatory system. Over time, especially with hypertension, this branch point can be a cause of concern on the part of physicians because it is an area that can develop **artery-clogging plaque.** In extreme cases, surgery may be needed to correct this problem.

Some may wonder how the heart contracts. In other words, what is the driving force that compels the heart to beat? The heart contracts when an electrical signal spreads through the heart in an orderly fashion. As a portion of the heart encounters the electoral impulse, that section contracts. The electrical signal responsible for the heartbeat originates within the heart in an area of the right atrium called the **sinoatrial node** (SA node). The SA node is sometimes called the "pacemaker" because it has the fastest rate (usually 60–100 bpm) of contraction and sets the pace that the rest of the heart follows. When the signal spreads outward from the SA node, it soon encounters an area called the **atrioventricular node** (AV node), which is also found in the right atrium. The AV node allows the electrical signal to pass through the heart's chambers in an orderly fashion and prevents the chambers from contracting at the same time. More specifically, when the electrical signal encounters the AV node, its speed slows down and it is redirected through the various nerve fibers that spread out over the ventricles (these are called **left and right bundle branches**, sometimes called the "Bundle of His"). These then lead to other pathways called **Purkinje fibers** that further transmit the electrical signal over the ventricles. In this way, the electoral signal is conducted in such a way that the heart beats in a uniform fashion.

Signal Pathway within the Heart

The electrical signal that stimulates heart contraction takes this path:

1. SA node starts the signal. The signal then travels to:
2. The AV node. From there, the signal goes to:
3. Left and right bundle branches. Then it goes to:
4. Purkinje fibers. From the Purkinje fibers, the signal makes contact with individual heart cells called **cardiocytes.**

Blood Flow to the Organs

While all organs receive blood, the flow of the blood to various organs is restricted under some circumstances (such as exercise, for example). But how does the blood know where to go? Basically, blood goes where it is needed most. This is accomplished by complex interactions among the blood vessels, the nervous system, and various chemical messengers that all work together. For example, with exercise, a large percentage of blood is directed to the exercising muscles. In this instance, less blood goes to the digestive system. Both the **parasympathetic** and **sympathetic** divisions of the autonomic nervous system send signals that expand and constrict blood vessels. Some of these impulses cause blood vessels to constrict (called **vasoconstriction**), which increases the resistance to blood flow. Other impulses cause blood vessels to expand (called **vasodilatation**). This increases blood flow to an area.

Some reading these words may be familiar with the amino acid arginine, which is metabolized into a gas called **nitric oxide** (NO). Nitric oxide is a potent vasodilator that might improve some symptoms of heart disease in older individuals.[37] Because of its vasodilatory effects, some fitness enthusiasts may experiment with "NO-boosting supplements" in the hopes of speeding recovery, improving strength, or enhancing the "pumped" look of muscles following exercise. Most of these claims, however, are more hype than science.[38] Conversely, compounds that act as vasoconstrictors include thromboxane and epinephrine (adrenalin).

So how does the brain "know" when blood pressure changes? **Baroreceptors** are specialized pressure receptors within blood vessels that monitor blood pressure changes and relay the information to the brain. Baroreceptors are found in the aortic arch as well as in the carotid arteries. They are sensitive to blood pressure changes and constantly relay information back to the brain.

Measuring Pulse

You may have measured your pulse during exercise by lightly feeling the carotid artery on the side of your neck. While this may work for you, it is usually not appropriate to do in other people. If you press too hard on the neck, you activate the baroreceptors in the carotid artery, which reduces heart rate. This will result in an inaccurate measurement of a person's RHR and THR calculations using the Karvonen formula. For better results, measure RHR at the **radial pulse,** which is located on the thumb side of the wrist.

Blood Pressure and the Heart

Blood pressure and the heart are intimately related. In fact, blood pressure is the result of the heart pumping blood through the blood vessels. When the heart beats, it pushes blood out of the heart. This results in the **systolic blood pressure.** When the heart fills with blood, before it contracts again, this results in the **diastolic pressure.** Thus, the blood pressure that you measure is the combination of two separate pressures—systolic and diastolic blood pressures—written as a fraction. The systolic is the top number of the fraction, while the diastolic pressure is the bottom. For example, if your blood pressure was 122/75, the systolic BP is 122 and 75 is the diastolic BP.

With aerobic exercise, the systolic BP tends to increase as exercise intensity increases. The diastolic BP, on the other hand, usually remains constant or decreases by a point or so. For example, the increase in BP might look like this: 120/80, 135/80, 150/80 and so on. With respect to resistance training, both systolic and diastolic blood pressure can increase dramatically, especially if combined with the **Valsalva effect**. In fact, blood pressures greater than 355/281 have been measured with strength training! However BP tends to return to normal shortly after cessation of exercise or before the next set is performed.[74]

When working with clients who have heart, kidney, or blood pressure issues, it is wise to measure blood pressure before and after exercise. This can tell you not only how the exercise program you have designed is affecting the client, but can also provide valuable information on whether or not they should exercise to begin with. Specifically, people whose resting blood pressure is greater than or equal to **200/115 mmHg** or close to this level should not exercise.[1] Rather, they should be referred to their physician, who can then take the appropriate action.

Blood Pressure Guidelines[75]

<120/80	Normal
120/80–139/89	Prehypertension
≥140/90	Hypertension

Notice that blood pressures of 120/80 are not called "normal" any longer. Technically, less than 120/80 is normal. A BP of 120/80 is now referred to as **prehypertension** or "pre high blood pressure." This change was made in light of evidence finding that in men age 55 years and older who started out with a BP of 120/80 appear to have a 90% chance of developing high blood pressure at some point in their lives.[75] So is 120/80 "normal" or is it really a prelude to high blood pressure? Everyone should know his or her blood pressure. Hypertension can lead to stroke—the 4th leading cause of death in the US.

Rate Pressure Product

The rate pressure product, also called, **double product**, is equal to the heart rate multiplied by the systolic blood pressure and is a factor used by medical professionals to estimate how much oxygen the heart is using. In other words, it measures how hard the heart is working. When either heart rate, systolic blood pressure, or both are elevated, as with exercise, the heart works harder. In healthy people who exercise regularly, rate pressure product is generally lower because exercise can lower resting heart rate and/or systolic blood pressure. Thus, when taken at rest, a lower rate pressure product usually means that the exercise-trained heart does not have to work as hard.

Heart Attack Warning Signs[156]

Constant or intermittent discomfort in the middle of the chest*	Shortness of breath*	Cold sweats
Jaw pain*	Nausea and/or vomiting*	Back pain*
Neck pain	Lightheadedness	Pain in one or both arms

* Common warning signs in women

Stroke Warning Signs[156]

Sudden numbness or weakness in face, arm or leg, particularly on one side of the body only	Sudden confusion or trouble speaking or understanding	Sudden trouble seeing in one or both eyes
Sudden trouble walking	Sudden loss of balance or coordination	Sudden headache with no known cause

How the Nervous System Affects Heart Rate

If the SA node usually sets the rhythm of the heart by beating between 60–100 bpm, how is it possible that people can have heart rates lower and higher than this? For example, depending on the age of the person, during exercise it is possible to have heart rates of 150 bpm or more! This is where the nervous system comes into play.

The **central nervous system** (CNS) consists of the brain and spinal cord. An extension of the CNS is the **peripheral nervous system** (PNS), which includes the nerves that stimulate organ systems outside of the brain and spinal cord, such as the arms, legs, abdominals, and even the heart.

The PNS can be divided into two parts: the **sympathetic** nervous system and the **parasympathetic** nervous system. This may sound confusing, but in reality it is not. The sympathetic nervous system speeds up heart rate, while the parasympathetic nervous system slows it down. Think of them like your car's accelerator pedal. When you press down on the accelerator, the car goes faster—this is what the sympathetic nervous system does. When you take your foot off of the accelerator, the car slows down—this is analogous to the function of the parasympathetic nervous system.

It is well known that people who exercise regularly have lower resting heart rates than non-exercisers. The reason for this is that, in those who work out regularly, the parasympathetic nervous system exerts greater control over the heart rate, causing RHR to decrease.

Sympathetic vs. Parasympathetic Nervous System[*]

Sympathetic Nervous System	Parasympathetic Nervous System
Mobilizes energy in times of stress	Control of sex
Increases heart rate	Conserves energy during times of rest
Increases force of muscle contractions	Decreases blood pressure
Reroutes blood to working muscles, away from digestive system	Decreases breathing rate
Increases glucose levels in blood	Stimulates digestion

*Not a complete list

How Well Is Your Heart Pumping?

While the interaction of the heart with exercise is complex, personal trainers should be familiar with a few heart-related concepts so that that they can interact intelligently with other health professionals and better explain to their clients some of the changes that occur when one undertakes a regular exercise program.

One of the factors is the **stroke volume** (SV), which is the amount of blood pumped out of the heart (specifically, from the left ventricle) per heartbeat. Each time the heart beats, it squirts out some blood. That amount is simply called the stroke volume. Technically, the stroke volume is also defined by the equation SV = EDV – ESV. End systolic volume (ESV) is the volume of blood in the heart after it has contracted (systole). End diastolic volume (EDV) is the amount of blood contained inside the left ventricle at the end of its filling phase (diastole). Another way of saying this is that EDV is the amount of blood in the heart just before it contracts. This gives rise to the other name for EDV—**preload**. In other words, it is the amount of blood with which the heart is "loaded" with before it contracts. As preload increases, stroke volume also increases.

Just as air stretches a balloon when you inflate it, the volume of blood inside the heart prior to contraction also exerts a stretching force on the heart walls. A greater volume of blood in the heart yields a greater stretch force—and also the greater recoil force as the heart contracts. This rubber band-recoil-like effect of the heart adds to its ability to eject blood and is referred to as the **Frank-Starling Law of the Heart**, named in honor of the two scientists who first described this effect. In essence, this law says that the more blood that fills the heart before it contracts, the greater the volume of blood ejected from the heart. This, in turn, allows each heartbeat to deliver more blood to the cardiovascular system and is another reason why we are able to exercise at higher intensities. Remember preload described above? Well, there is also afterload. **Afterload** describes how hard it is to eject blood from the heart. In order for blood to leave the heart, the pressure of the blood in the left ventricle must be greater than the overall blood pressure. If the pressure outside the heart is greater than that inside the heart, less blood is ejected. This reduces not only cardiac output and stroke volume, but overall health as well. High blood pressure (hypertension) is a condition that can increase afterload. Holding breath during weight lifting (Valsalva maneuver) also increases afterload and can lead to one losing consciousness.

Another heart-related term is the **ejection fraction**. As stated previously, some blood remains inside the left ventricle after the heart contracts—this is normal. If we could measure the amount of blood within the left ventricle before it contracted (the end diastolic volume) and compare that to the amount that was ejected (stroke volume), we would get a fraction called the ejection fraction. Another way of saying this is that the ejection fraction is the percentage of the blood that is actually ejected from the left ventricle of the heart compared to what was in the left ventricle before it contracted. Normally, the heart ejects between 55–0% of the blood in the left ventricle with each heartbeat. Exercise-trained hearts have even greater ejection fractions. In fact, in highly trained athletes, the ejection fraction might be more than 90%. In people who have heart disease, ejection might be only 30%. Mathematically, ejection fraction can be calculated from two different-looking yet identical equations:

$$EF = SV/EDV \quad \text{and} \quad EF = \frac{EDV - ESV}{EDV}$$

EF is ejection fraction, SV is stroke volume, EDV is end diastolic volume, and ESV is end systolic volume.

Cardiac output is the amount of blood pumped from the heart (from the left ventricle) in one minute. In some textbooks, it is abbreviated as "CO" or "Q." Cardiac output is determined by multiplying the heart rate times the stroke volume. This gives rise to the classic equation: CO = HR x SV. Thus, as heart rate and stroke volume increase, cardiac output also increases.

During exercises performed in an upright position like running, walking, or cycling, cardiac output increases because both stroke volume and heart rate increase.[29] As can be seen through stroke volume and the ejection fraction, those who exercise on a regular basis tend to have greater cardiac outputs than non-exercisers.

Obviously, fitness trainers will probably not be calculating stroke volumes, ejection fractions, or cardiac outputs. The equations are presented to help give you a better understanding of these concepts and to help you explain them to clients if the need arises. Sometimes fitness professionals may find themselves interacting with other members of the health care system like physicians, chiropractors, and nurses. Knowledge of these and other concepts discussed in this book goes a long way in establishing yourself as a professional member of their team.

Blood Flow during Exercise

Blood is the source of oxygen and nutrients, making blood a valuable currency. Just as you might allocate your money to pay different bills, so does the body. During exercise, the body automatically redistributes blood flow such that the muscles and organ systems that are participating in exercise get the most blood, while those muscles and organ systems that are not receive a reduced blood flow.

Acute Changes from CV Exercise

Acute changes refer to short-term changes that occur soon after exercise begins. In other words, these occur after you have been working out for a few seconds to many minutes. Before you even enter the gym, your heart rate begins to increase. This is the body's way of preparing itself for exercise. Related to this, stroke volume, ejection fraction, and cardiac output also increase during exercise.

One of the first changes with exercise occurs within the blood vessels just under the skin, where a vasodilation (opening up) of the vessels occurs, allowing blood to come close to the skin's surface to give off excess heat. In this way, the body helps to cool itself during exercise.

Blood flow to the muscles changes as well. Specifically, muscle blood flow tends to be about 15–20% of cardiac output at rest but with exercise may increase to as much as 75% for most people and as much as 90% in some elite athletes.[41] This occurs because blood travels to locations where it is needed most. Conversely, blood flow to organs such as the stomach usually diminishes during exercise.

As for blood pressure, remember that systolic blood pressure tends to increase as exercise intensity increases. Diastolic blood pressure, on the other hand, either remains constant or decreases a little.

Some hormones also change with exercise. As you exercise, your cells use glucose to help power exercising muscles. **Glucagon**, a hormone made in the pancreas, raises blood sugar. Glucagon begins to increase during exercise. With respect to insulin, it tends to reduce during exercise. This may seem backward to some because insulin is needed for sugar (glucose) to be used by the cells of the body. However, during exercise, the body is more efficient at using insulin. This is because exercise causes the number **insulin receptors** to increase on the surface of the body cells. More insulin receptors means greater glucose extraction without the need for extra insulin. Also, when we exercise, we ramp up the use of non-insulin-dependent sugar gateways. These gateways do not need insulin to work. Thus, by becoming more efficient at using insulin and activating alternate pathways for glucose to enter the cells, the body does not need as much insulin during exercise. As you might guess, this has important implications for addressing diabetes. For more on exercise and diabetes, see my blog post, "Can Type II Diabetes Be Cured?" at Joe-Cannon.com.

Epinephrine (adrenaline) made in the adrenal glands is another hormone that helps boost glucose levels and heart rate. It also increases overall alertness and assists with fat metabolism. Epinephrine tends to increase during exercise and also produces more forceful muscle contractions.

Growth hormone (GH) increases during exercise, especially in untrained people. Growth hormone impacts a range of body systems, including immune function and muscle growth.

Summary: Effects of an Acute Bout of Aerobic Exercise*

Parameter	Exercise Effect
Heart rate	Increases before exercise begins. Increases also as exercise intensity increases.
Stroke volume, ejection fraction, cardiac output	All increase with increasing exercise intensities.
Blood flow to skin	Increases to help dissipate heat; blood flow to working muscles increases; decreased flow to "non-priority" organ systems.
Blood pressure	Systolic increases; diastolic remains constant or decreases slightly.
Glucagon	Increases.
Insulin	Decreases. Cell sensitivity to insulin increases.
Epinephrine	Increases.
Growth hormone	Increases.

* Not a complete list

Chronic Adaptations from CV Exercise

Chronic (long-term) aerobic exercise results in several adaptations. Below are just a few of the positive adaptations associated with long-term aerobic exercise.

One of the most dramatic changes is that regular exercise tends to reduce the risk of dying from all major diseases.[1] The amount of exercise thought to be sufficient for this purpose varies from expert to expert but is generally 30–60 minutes performed most days of the week. One study noted that just 15 minutes of walking per day not only reduced mortality but also increased average lifespan by 3 years.[187]

Between 2–10 weeks after starting to workout, a decrease resting heart rate (RHR) may occur.[27] This decrease in RHR is thought to be the result of an increase in parasympathetic nervous activity coupled with a decrease in the influence of the sympathetic nervous system. In addition, the heart rate during submaximal exercise (less than an all-out effort) is lower as well. This occurs because the heart becomes stronger with exercise training. Thus, what would once have over-stressed the heart in the past no longer does so.

The heart grows a bit larger with exercise. Not only do the chambers of the heart increase in size, but the thickness of the heart muscle itself does as well. This is especially true of the muscle of the left ventricle, the main pumping chamber of the heart.[42]

After exercise, heart rate returns to normal more quickly.[42] This is sometimes referred to as the **heart rate recovery time**. Returning to normal rapidly is usually indicative of a healthier heart. A longer recovery time may indicate a greater risk of dying from heart disease, even in otherwise healthy people. According to one study, the heart rate should decrease by at least 12 beats within the first minute after strenuous exercise.[189]

Regular aerobic exercise stimulates the body to ramp up its blood production. Specifically, not only are more red blood cells made, but the watery, fluid part of blood (plasma) also increases in volume. This increase in blood volume means more blood enters and leaves the heart with each beat.

Capillaries are the smallest blood vessels in the body. In the capillaries, oxygen and nutrients pass from the blood into the cells. Long-term aerobic exercise results in an increase in capillary density, and this increase is greatest in the muscles that are participating in the exercise.[28] In other words, if you were a runner, we would expect to see increased capillary density in the legs. Other research suggests that the capillaries within the heart itself also increase following aerobic endurance exercise.[43] This suggests that the heart may be better at absorbing oxygen and nutrients.

In some studies, blood pressure has been shown to decrease following long-term aerobic exercise.[1] Specifically, both systolic and diastolic blood pressure might decrease following exercise training.[30] This effect seems to be greatest in people with hypertension.[30]

Scientists can estimate which macronutrient (fat, carbohydrate, or protein) the body is primarily using by measuring the amounts of oxygen and carbon dioxide inhaled and exhaled. This gives rise to the **respiratory exchange ratio** (RER). Mathematically, RER is equal to the volume of carbon dioxide exhaled divided by the volume of oxygen inhaled.[42] Another way of saying this is that RER = VCO2/VO2. Mathematics aside, an RER of 1.00 means that you are burning all of your energy from carbohydrates; an RER of about 0.7 means that you are burning all of your energy from fat. An RER of about 0.82 means that you are burning all protein. At rest RER falls somewhere between 0.7 and 1.0, meaning that we generally burn a mixture of fats and carbohydrates. In fact, we tend to burn a little more fat than carbohydrate at rest. It also turns out that after several months of exercise training, RER decreases during exercise at submaximal levels (i.e., it moves closer to 0.7). This means that exercise-trained people burn fat more efficiently than those who do not exercise regularly. As a personal trainer, it is unlikely that you will ever calculate RER. However, remembering RER numbers can be valuable if your career path leads you toward working with athletes, in the weight loss field, or in advanced exercise testing.

Many studies find that exercise can help reduce total cholesterol and LDL ("bad cholesterol") as well as raise HDL ("good cholesterol").[30, 31] Levels of triglycerides have also been shown to reduce following exercise training.[30] These results have been in observed in both men and women. While the usual recommendations call for at least 30 minutes of continuous aerobic exercise on most days of the week, some research also suggests that splitting exercise into smaller blocks of time appears to promote similar benefits to that of continuous exercise.[32, 33] This can be useful for people with busy schedules. Studies show the moderate levels of exercise training can help improve the immune system.[45] Exhaustive exercise (i.e., running a marathon), however, is associated with decreased immunity.[44]

One often neglected adaptation involves the body's own antioxidant defense systems. Clients may be under the assumption that antioxidants can only be obtained from dietary supplements. The body has an array of internal antioxidant defenses that help protect us from free radicals. These defenses include enzymes like **superoxide dismutase (SOD)**, **catalase** and **glutathione peroxidase**. Exercise can increase many of these enzymes and probably other defenses as well.[34]

Summary: Effects of Long-Term Aerobic Exercise*

Parameter	How Exercise Helps
Death from all causes	Risk decreases
Resting heart rate	Tends to lower
Submaximal exercise heart rate	Tends to lower
Overall heart size	Tends to enlarge somewhat
Muscles of left ventricle	Tend to enlarge and grow stronger
Blood	Increase in RBCs, hemoglobin, and plasma
Stroke volume, ejection fraction, and cardiac output	All tend to increase
Capillary density of working muscles	Tends to increase
Heart capillary density	Tends to increase
Blood pressure	Both systolic & diastolic tend to lower, especially in those with high blood pressure
Cholesterol, LDL, & triglycerides	Tends to be reduced
Ability to burn fat (RER)	Greater ability to burn fat
HDL	Tends to increase
Immunity	Improved with moderate levels of exercise
Body's antioxidant defense systems	Tends to increase

* Not a complete list

Chapter 8

DESIGNING EXERCISE PROGRAMS

This chapter reviews many of the basic and essential tools and concepts with which fitness trainers need to be familiar when designing an exercise program. While not specifically covered in this chapter, it should be understood that, ideally, before any exercise program can be developed, the client should first undergo some form of fitness testing to determine weak or strong areas and to complete the necessary paperwork to enable the trainer to gauge the health and training experience of the individual.

Principles of Training

The following are principles or laws of exercise and are important to be familiar with, as they will help guide whatever decisions you make with regard to putting together an exercise program for a client or for yourself.

Principle of Individual Differences

This principle takes into account our innate genetic differences and basically says that not everyone will get the same results from an exercise program. Muscle fiber type, bone density, anabolic hormones, tendon placement, and VO₂max all have genetic influences that may either enhance or hinder results. Thus, two people following the same exercise program may not achieve identical results because of differences in their genetic makeup.

Principle of Specificity

This principle basically says that a training program should usually progress from very general to very specific exercises. For beginners, an overall basic program that is not very specific is best. As fitness improves, it is possible to target exercise to meet their individual needs and goals. Another definition for this principle states that if your goal is to be better at some specific task, then you have to do that task if it is to improve. This gives rise to the phrase "specific adaptations to imposed demands," or the **SAID Principle**. While this may sound complicated, it is not. Basically, it means that if you want to be a better runner, then run. If you want to be better at the bench press, do the bench press. The body will respond *specifically* to those exercise *demands* that are *imposed* upon it. To illustrate, I once met with an 80-year-old woman who told me that she could lift 130 pounds on the seated leg press, yet when she accidentally slipped and fell, she discovered she was unable to get up from the floor. She was not hurt from the fall, but she was just not strong enough. This made sense, because the leg press, while working many of the same muscles that she would use when rising from the floor, is not the same thing as actually getting up from the floor. After a few weeks of practice, she was able to get up from the floor unassisted.

Principle of Progressive Overload

This principle states that no positive change occurs unless the body is overloaded a little beyond its level of comfort. For example, if you could lift 100 pounds 10 times and you wanted to be stronger, then you would need to increase the load lifted to 105 pounds. You may not be able to lift it 10 times at first, but eventually you will be able to do so.

We overload the body by manipulating one or more of four factors that are collectively called the **FITT Principle**. In essence, the FITT Principle is what makes up the overload principle. "FITT" stands for:

> * **Frequency of exercise.** For example, increasing exercise from 2 days a week to 3 days a week.
> * **Intensity of exercise.** For example, increasing the weight lifted from 100 pounds to 105 pounds or increasing the speed on the treadmill from 3 mph to 3.2 mph.
> * **Time of exercise.** For example, increasing your time in the gym from 30 minutes to 40 minutes. Here is a tip for trainers: If you ever deal with a person who has a special need like someone who has high blood pressure, remember that increasing the time of exercise is usually safer than increasing the intensity of exercise.
> * **Type of exercise.** An example of this would be moving from strength training machines to free weights or for bodyweight exercises to machines.

Principle of Maintenance

According to this principle, once you are at the fitness level that you desire to achieve, continue to train at that level to maintain what you have achieved.

Principle of Adaptation

Eventually the body will adapt the exercise stimulus. Things that used to be difficult are not anymore. To continue to progress, the routine must be altered somehow (see FITT principle above).

Principle of Disuse or Reversibility

This is often called the "use it or lose it principle." If you do not continue to exercise, you will eventually lose all of the benefits that you obtained in the first place. Depending on fitness level, it is possible to begin to atrophy after 2 weeks of not training.

Warm-Up

Generally, a warm-up consists of 5–10 minutes of light aerobic activity. Calisthenics can also be used if they are of sufficient length. The goal of the warm-up is to prepare the body for the exercise program. This is sometimes referred to as a **general warm-up.** The benefits of warming up are many and include:[1]

1. Increased metabolic rate above resting levels
2. Improved reaction time
3. Improved flexibility
4. Possible reduced risk of injury during exercise

5. Possible reductions in heart rhythm abnormalities (e.g., heart attack)

One may also choose to perform an **exercise-specific warm-up**. For example, one may perform a few sets of a bench press at a low resistance prior to going heavy. For safety reasons, it is best to perform a general warm-up before doing an exercise-specific warm-up. It is also important to note that stretching usually does not constitute a good warm-up because most people do not stretch long enough.

Stretching and Injuries

Contrary to popular belief, the act of stretching just prior to exercise does not appear to significantly reduce the frequency of sports-related injuries.[103] However, some research suggests that regular stretching may offer a mild protective effect.[104] Likewise, stretching before exercise does not appear to significantly reduce delayed onset muscle soreness (DOMS).[103, 104] While static stretching is often advised for most people, an argument can be made for dynamic stretching in athletes because of the forceful nature of those events.

Classifying Types of Exercises

Personal trainers usually make a distinction between exercises on the basis of how much muscle they recruit. This leads to the classifications called multi-joint and single-joint exercises. A **multi-joint exercise** is one that enlists large muscle groups. Squats, bench presses, and push-ups are examples of multi-joint exercises. Multi-joint exercises are also sometimes called **core exercises** because they form the basis or core of a strength training program. Another term also used is **compound exercise**. "Compound" refers to the fact that multi-joint movements result from the interaction of a number of muscle groups. In contrast, a **single-joint exercise** is one that uses fewer muscles. Biceps curls and triceps extensions are examples of this. While both types of exercises are essential, those that are multi-joint are usually seen as being more important because they tend to be more sports-specific and better mimic one's ADLs.

Another way to classify exercises is to use the terms **open chain** and **closed chain**. Consider a chain that you wear around your neck. If the chain is broken, the ends are free to dangle. An open chain exercise is one in which the feet (or hands) are freely moving (e.g., leg extension). In contrast, a closed chain exercise is one in which the feet (or hands) are stabilized on the floor or other surface and do not move (e.g., leg press). One can think of closed chain as being somewhat similar to multi-joint movements, while open chain are somewhat analogous to single-joint movements.

Exercise Sequence

Let us review some logical rules to remember when designing a program. Of course, there are exceptions to almost every rule, but following these basic guidelines will help when you design a program for your clients.

- ➤ **Warm-up should occur first.** The warm-up can help reduce injury.
- ➤ **Large muscle groups before small muscle groups.** In general, work the legs, chest, and back before the biceps, triceps, and other small muscle groups. Multi-joint exercises usually come before single-joint movements. Working the smaller muscles first to "pre-exhaust" them is an advanced technique that should be reserved only for advanced lifters.
- ➤ **Do not train the same muscles maximally 2 days in a row.** Remember, muscles become stronger after exercise. Training the same muscle without enough rest may decrease these benefits and increase risk for injury. Generally, 24–48 hours is recommended between strength training sessions. Depending on fitness level, the difficulty of the routine, and the age of the individual, even more time may be required.
- ➤ **Power movements should be placed early in the workout.** In other words, do the hardest exercises at the beginning of a workout. It is very difficult to exert maximal power, so it is safer to do so when the client is feeling strongest. Do not wait until the end of the workout when they are tired.
- ➤ **Skill- and agility-related movements should be placed early in the workout.** Movements that require balance, a special skill, or hand/eye coordination should be performed early. Again, put the hardest movements at the beginning. Depending on the fitness level of the individual, even walking could be considered a skill- or agility-related movement.
- ➤ **Work the abs and low back *after* working muscle groups that involve the abs or low back.** Fatiguing the abs or low back first can reduce their ability to help stabilize the trunk during multi-joint activities, which might increase injury risk.
- ➤ **Work the muscles that you want to most heavily emphasize early in the workout.** Suppose that you want to focus on the shoulders. Because the client is strongest at the start of the workout, movements that emphasize shoulders would be some of the first muscles targeted. This is for advanced lifters only.
- ➤ **Perform new exercises early.** Any new activities that you teach a client should be placed early in the workout to reduce the risk of injury. After he or she masters the new activity, it can be put in its proper place.
- ➤ **Progress from machines to free weights.** Machines are usually easier to use, so starting a client with these may be safer. Some trainers might prefer to teach body weight exercises first and then machines or free weights. Consider what is best and safest for the client.
- ➤ **Do free weights *before* machines if both are performed in the same workout.** Because machines are usually easier, leaving them until last, in theory, reduces injury while still letting the muscle group to be worked.
- ➤ **Cool down.** This is the reversal of the warm-up. Cooling down returns the body to its pre-exercise state, can prevent dizziness after exercise, and may even help stabilize heart function.[1]
- ➤ **Stretch.** Stretching after the workout may be more efficient and effective than stretching before exercise and appears to confer the same benefits.[183]
- ➤ **First increase the number of repetitions, then increase the number of sets before increasing amount of weight.** Following this guideline will give the body time to *adapt* to the rigors of exercise and reduce the risk of injury.

Abs Every Day?

The rationale for working the abdominal muscles every day stems from the high concentration of slow-twitch, type I fibers found in the abdominal area. These fibers are geared toward endurance and recover faster than type II fibers. Those who say that training abs every other day is best usually base their argument on the fact that during a crunch or sit-up, one is lifting about 50–60% of his or her body weight. This is somewhat analogous to lifting weights, and the guideline for that is to perform similar exercises every other day. So who is right? Both arguments have merit. However, consider the client and his or her fitness level when making this decision. Unfit people or novices are best served by working the abdominals every other day, as this will reduce DOMS and injuries. For more fit people, every day may be ok, but to be safe, try different types of abdominal exercises that work not only the rectus abdominis but also the other muscles of the abdominal region. Remember, abdominal exercises alone will not create a "six-pack." That comes from good genetics, aerobic exercise, and eating fewer calories.

Designing Exercise Programs

All exercise programs (strength or cardio) can be said to have the following stages: initial conditioning stage, improvement stage, and maintenance stage.

The **initial conditioning stage** is the point in the program when the body first becomes accustomed to the rigors of regular exercise. During this phase, a primary goal should be to establish a foundation on which to base more difficult future training sessions. For many clients, this means improving muscle endurance and cardiovascular endurance. Other goals should be to bolster confidence, foster a healthy lifestyle, and develop a love for working out. Now is not the time to overwhelm someone with multiple sets or produce large degrees of muscle soreness (DOMS). Depending on fitness level, this stage may last for 4–8 weeks and possibly up to 12 weeks.

The **improvement stage** occurs after the initial conditioning stage and is when the exercise stimulus is gradually increased to foster further improvements. Resistance used, as well as intensity of aerobic activity are ramped up. These modifications should only be made according to the client's individual needs, wants, and health history. This stage might last for 4–6 months.

Some people may eventually reach a point where they are happy and do not want or need to progress any further. This **maintenance stage** is where the client basically maintains the fitness level that he or she has developed up to this point. This may also be a good time to establish new, attainable goals or to tweak the program to keep it from getting boring.

When putting together a strength training program, it is important to have an idea of the basic principles behind achieving various goals. For example, someone desiring muscular hypertrophy should be trained differently than someone looking to improve muscular endurance. Also, a program for a beginner will be less intense than that for someone who has been working out for several years.

Now that we have reviewed the major stages of an exercise program, let us return to the initial conditioning stage and review basic guidelines that should be followed when working with beginners.

Working Out: The First 8–12 Weeks

One of the first things that we notice when babies learn to walk is that they fall down frequently. Some may assume that this happens because their muscles are not yet strong enough. While this is partially true, there is another reason why this happens.

Learning a new exercise or exercise program requires not only that the muscles, ligaments, and tendons grow stronger, but also that alterations take place in the brain and nervous system. These are referred to as **neurological changes**. When you first begin to do something new, whether it is jogging, lifting weights, or bowling, your nervous system is inexperienced at the task and does not yet know how to coordinate your muscles in the way that produces the best or most efficient movement pattern—it is as if your brain and muscles speak different languages. To help them communicate, changes must be made within the brain and nervous system such that the muscles can come to understand what is being said to them.

In the gym, it is easy to see who has not yet acquired the necessary neurological changes for performing exercises efficiently. Look at the people who are doing a bench press with a barbell. If they wobble the barbell back and forth as they lift the weight and it looks like one arm is lifting the weight more quickly than the other, that is a usually dead give-away that they are new to the exercise. With respect to children, most gains in strength before puberty are due to neurological changes. In adults, on the other hand, it generally it takes about 8–12 weeks for these neurological changes to kick in, but this can vary depending on the age of the person and how difficult the exercise is.

Programs for Beginners

It is safe to say that many people hire fitness trainers because they are not sure how to safely improve their fitness and health. They want guidance. They also want results, and more often than not, they want those results quickly. This creates a dilemma for the trainer because achieving fast results—especially with beginners—usually goes hand in hand with increased injury. In turn, injury limits the client's ability to train and reduces the ability of the trainer to earn a living. It also increases the odds that the trainer will develop a bad reputation. Fitness professionals should be just that—*professionals*. When faced with a person who has never worked out or who has done so infrequently, yet wants a magazine-cover body in a few weeks or months, the trainer should help the person understand that this is unlikely. They should then progress the client slowly to reduce injury risk. Programs for beginners need not be strenuous or overly lengthy in order to be effective. In fact, it is possible to work the entire body effectively in as little as 20–30 minutes. Most beginners do not need to work out more than 2–3 times per week.

When designing an exercise program for a beginner, remember that while the muscles may quickly grow stronger, the tendons, ligaments, and other connective tissues will take longer. This is why trying to achieve quick results often results in injury. Because of this, novices are best suited with single-set programs that use low resistance and relatively high numbers of repetitions for the first few months.[107] Remember that for the first several weeks, many of the improvements that they see are due to neurological factors. In other words, it is not so much that the muscles are getting stronger but rather that the central nervous system is communicating more effectively with the muscles. A better mind-body connection allows for better coordination of muscle recruitment and efficiency in lifting. Let us now discuss this in terms of weight, sets and repetitions.

Why Are Training Sessions 30 Minutes?

At some health clubs, personal training sessions are limited to about 30 minutes. There are several reasons why this is so. First, most beginners lack the endurance (and desire) to work out for much longer than this. Second, 30 minutes is often the minimum amount of exercise experts recommend for overall health. Third, some research notes greater dropout rates when workouts last more than 1 hour.[188] Unfortunately, some trainers desiring to give the client the best workout possible may opt to use advanced routines like super sets. This increases DOMS and the risk of injury. Since the majority of clients are beginners, the most time efficient and safest way to train them is to do circuit training.

How much weight and how many repetitions should be used? Novices are best suited with relatively light resistances. However, one does not want to lift a weight so many times that injury results. There is no perfect resistance to use with beginners because everybody has different abilities. Thus, it is best to choose a weight that can be lifted safely and comfortably 12–20 times. Some fitness trainers may also choose to make this a "12–20 RM," where RM stands for "repetition maximum." Repetition maximum represents the most weight that a person can lift safely a certain number of times with good lifting technique. For example, a weight that is equal to 12 RM can only be lifted 12 times with good lifting technique. Determining RM usually means performing multiple sets to obtain the load that one is seeking. For the untrained person, this will probably lead to significant DOMS. Thus, for novices, determining RM may not always be necessary.

Another alternative is to determine the load by using the **RPE scale**. Suppose the person is to perform 12 repetitions. Choose a weight that you feel is appropriate and ask the person how heavy it feels on a scale from 0 to 10, where 10 is a super heavy weight and 0 is extremely easy. Ask them how heavy it feels when they first lift the weight, half way through the set, and again at the end of the set. This will give you an idea of how they feel during the entire set. For people with special needs (e.g., arthritis) you may want the intensity to be about 2–3 on the RPE scale, while for a healthy person, 5–6 may be appropriate. Everyone is different, and as the trainer, your job is to pick an intensity that emphasizes benefits while minimizing risks. While the RPE scale may not be 100% accurate, with novices, you do not need to be overly precise. The goal is to get them accustomed to lifting weights, boost their confidence, and most importantly, minimize injury.

For beginners, 8–12 repetitions for healthy persons under 50 years of age and 10–15 repetitions for those older than 50–60 years of age are generally recommend.[1] However, for very untrained persons, lifting a weight for only 8 repetitions may be too much. Also, these guidelines are not significantly different than the general guideline of 12–20 repetitions mentioned above. Generally, the greater the number of repetitions, the more muscular endurance is improved, while with lower repetitions, more strength is gained. For beginners, improvement of strength should not be the primary concern (even though it may be the client's). Instead, the trainer should focus on preparing the client's body for the more difficult training to come in the future. For most people, this is best accomplished with lighter loads. When in doubt, first increase the repetitions, then increase the sets, and then increase the weight lifted. Following this formula should progress people slowly enough that the nervous system, ligaments, and tendons have time to catch up to what the person is doing.

The number of sets to be completed per exercise is often a point of contention among trainers, with many believing that several sets (i.e., 2 sets or more) are superior to single-set programs. Many studies find that multiple sets are superior for improving strength and hypertrophy, but that does not mean that they are best for everyone. Factors that might necessitate only performing one set may include experience level, time constraints, and health issues. For healthy, sedentary people, the ACSM recommends one set of 8–12 exercises that target the major muscles of the body.[1] Also, single-set programs have been shown to increase strength in beginners for the at least the first 2–3 months of training.[107] After a few months, they may have adopted a healthy lifestyle and want to do more. Until that happens, single-set programs may serve the needs of the client best.

Benefits of One-Set Programs

Improves strength	Not boring	Easy to work whole body in a single session
Improves muscular endurance	Allows busy people to fit fitness into their lives	Safest for those with special needs
Reduces injury risk	Is time efficient	Greater degree of adherence for beginners

For programs requiring multiple sets, the rest periods between them will vary according to the person's goals, age, health concerns, and fitness level. A general guideline is that rest periods should range from 30 seconds to 2–5 minutes between sets. This is where the individualized nature of personal training comes into play. As a fitness professional, you will rely not only on what the client is telling you about how he or she feels, but also on what you observe as the individual performs each exercise. For example, a person may tell you that he or she feels fine and can do another set while you notice the arms shaking during each repetition and exercise technique breaking down. This tells you the person may have reached his or her threshold and needs additional rest between sets or needs to use a lower resistance.

Beginner Strength Program: Basic Guidelines

Resistance	Repetitions	Sets	Rest between sets	Workouts/wk
Light loads	12–20	1 set for first few months	30 sec to 2–5 min	2–3

Training Goal: Weight Loss

Many people hire personal trainers for weight loss help. Unfortunately, exercise alone will probably not help people lose weight. To be most effective, exercise must be combined with eating fewer calories per day. Check the calorie counter on the treadmill next time you work. You might notice that only 200 or so calories are used after 20 minutes of exercise. That is fewer calories than are in some protein bars. Thus, with the exception of huge amounts of activity (that many cannot or will not do), exercise alone will probably not lead to long-term weight reduction.

One reason why exercise alone will not work may be understood in terms of an individual's **24-hour energy expenditure.** Essentially, different factors cause us to burn calories over a 24-hour period. There are only three things that burn calories:

1. Resting metabolism
2. Exercise
3. Thermic effect of food

Of these three factors, resting metabolism burns the most calories (about 66%). Exercise (at best) only accounts for about 30% of daily calories used, and this percentage is even smaller in beginners. The other 10% comes from the calories used digesting food. Therefore, we actually burn the most calories when we are doing nothing.

Because exercise alone is unlikely to work, it needs to be combined with a reduction in calories. Weight loss guidelines usually call for a calorie deficit of between 500–1000 calories a day.[1] While this will likely work, eliminating this many calories may be challenging for some people. Other experts suggest that reducing calories by 300–400 calories per day may be optimal for women and men who are trying to lose fat without sacrificing metabolic rate.[113] Regardless, whatever one chooses, it is important to first determine an approximate number of calories currently consumed and reduce this by a subtle amount. Over time, any small reduction in calories will cause the body to use its stored fat and glycogen reserves, resulting in weight loss. Various fitness trackers, websites, and apps can help people track calories and exercise and may provide both insights and weight-loss motivation.

Some experts consider losing 10% of initial body weight to be a good starting point for weight loss.[1] For example, a client weighing 300 pounds should first attempt to lose 30 pounds. One might tackle this by breaking up 30 pounds into 5- or 10-pound increments. Reduce weight slowly, aiming for 0.5–2 pounds per week. This will help preserve muscle mass and maintain metabolic rate. Some research suggests that losing more than 0.5 pounds per week may slow metabolic rate.[157]

Some people may opt for a diet program to achieve weight loss. Most diets will probably cause short-term weight loss, especially those that restrict carbohydrate intake, as they promote glycogen breakdown and the release of water stored in the body. Remember that each gram of glycogen used releases about 3 grams of water. In other words, burning off one pound of glycogen releases 3 pounds of water! This is why one of the first signs of weight loss on low-carb diets is frequent urination. Interestingly, long-term weight loss from carbohydrate restriction does not appear to be superior to simply reducing calories.[114] When used over an extended period of time (>6 months), it appears that people on low-carb diets simply eat fewer calories out of boredom with the diet's food choices. One big problem with most diets is that the individual eventually goes off of the diet and returns to old eating habits, which usually results in a regaining of weight. For more on this phenomenon, see my blog post, "Low-Carb Diets: How They Really Work," available at Joe-Cannon.com.

By itself, dieting can lead to significant loss of muscle tissue, which is unhealthy. This is why dieting alone is usually not recommended. Exercise reduces this loss. It usually does not matter what form of exercise people choose—strength or cardiovascular training—as either will help. *The National Weight Control Registry* (www.NWCR.ws) has been tracking people who have been successful at losing weight and keeping it off. They report that 90% of the people in their registry exercise at least 60 minutes per day. As a general rule, activities should incorporate large muscle groups (i.e., the chest, back, and legs) to maximize calorie usage. Depending on individual needs and limitations, ADL-type activities may also be included to improve quality of life. Since boredom as well as lack of strength and endurance may be issues that come into play, circuit training may be most appropriate for these individuals. Adding in a bike or treadmill to the circuit will increase calorie use and enhance the aerobic aspect of the circuit. For those with joint issues, pool exercise may be particularly helpful. Keeping exercise intensity low will ensure that the deconditioned person can sustain at least 30 minutes of physical activity. When designing an exercise circuit, keep in mind that very large people may not easily fit into some strength machines.

Body Fat Testing: Yes or No?

The notion of performing body composition testing on people looking for weight loss is controversial in some circles. Some say to do it, as it will help spur the client toward future results when he or she sees what he or she has accomplished. Others say to refrain from doing it, as it may embarrass the client. Particularly in the case of body fat calipers, some clients may not like being touched by people whom they barely know, especially those of the opposite gender. Moreover, some tests may not even be accurate in those who are very overweight. Personally, if the test is warranted, I explain the benefits of body composition testing and let the client make the call. If the person says no, that is fine—he or she may change perspectives at some point after thinking it over. The big issue is that we never want to make another person feel uncomfortable. Presenting yourself in the most professional manner can go a long way toward making others feel at ease around you, which will help you help your clients experience greater success.

Training Goal: Muscular Endurance

Muscular endurance is defined as the ability of a muscle to exert force for extended periods of time and comes into play during activities ranging from carrying groceries to running triathlons. Strength training can improve muscular endurance and aerobic exercise performance. To improve muscular endurance, it is necessary to use lighter resistances, around 12–15 RM, and to perform 1–3 sets per exercise.[78] Thus, the intensity of exercise is generally low when training for muscle endurance. In addition, the rest periods should be short, generally less than 30 seconds between sets.[78] Short rest periods are needed because this most simulates endurance activities such as marathons. Training for this effect mainly taxes the aerobic (oxidative) energy system and type I muscle fibers.

Training Goal: Muscle Hypertrophy

When training for muscle size, the volume (weight x repetitions x sets) of exercise tends be greater than that for muscle endurance. In general, the resistance used should be between 8RM–12RM. Because heavier resistances are used, rest periods between sets tend to be longer, with 30–90 seconds being common.[78] One key concept here is to stress the muscle again before it has fully recovered.[181] As the person becomes more fit, less rest time may be required between sets. Moreover, performing one set may eventually not be enough to foster the results that the client seeks, and the number of sets will need to be increased.

Some research shows that hypertrophy training tends to elicit greater release in GH and testosterone compared with those designed to improve muscle strength only.[181] In addition, multiple exercises per body part appear to be better than single sets at producing hypertrophy.[76, 77] During hypertrophy, much metabolic stress is placed on the anaerobic energy system. These programs usually target both type I and type II fibers. While not normally discussed, it is possible for type I fibers to undergo some hypertrophy. However, the degree to which these fibers grow is less than that of type II fibers.[77]

Interestingly, the biochemical process by which hypertrophy occurs appears to be different for each fiber type. Specifically, type II fibers undergo hypertrophy mostly because of an increase in protein synthesis. Type I fibers, on the other hand, appear to grow because of a reduction in protein breakdown.[111] In addition, there is evidence that traditionally used bodybuilding programs tend to hypertrophy both type I and type II fibers. This is contrasted with that of power lifting, which seems to result in less type I fiber hypertrophy.[77] Hypertrophy-based programs almost certainly also promote the conversion of type IIb fibers into the more athletic type IIa fibers as well.

How Long before Hypertrophy Occurs?

People will often ask you how long it takes for muscles get bigger. In reality, the body responds to strength training after just a few workouts.[108] However, changes in muscle fiber cross sectional area and hypertrophy usually require at least 8 weeks of consistent training.[77]

Training Goal: Muscular Power vs. Muscular Strength

Muscular strength and muscular power are not the same thing. Strength is the exertion of force over time. Power, on the other hand, is basically explosive strength. Power packs a big punch but does not last long (i.e., no more than about 30 seconds). Nevertheless, the protocols to improve both power and strength are very similar. In general, improving strength or power requires very heavy weights (~1–8 RM) and comparatively long rest periods (2–5 minutes) between sets.[78] In its purest sense, power-oriented workouts recruit mostly the ATP/CP system, while strength-centered use mostly glycolysis and the ATP/CP systems. You can use the following tables as guidelines when training people. Remember, each person is different, so do not feel obligated to adhere to the loads, sets, and repetitions exactly as they appear here. For most clients, they are mere recommendations, not hard-and-fast rules.

Quick Reference: Basic Guidelines for Different Goals[5]

	Load (% of 1RM)	Repetitions	Sets	Rest	Volume
Endurance	≤67%	12–20	2–3	<30 sec	Medium
Hypertrophy	67 to 85%	6–12	3–6	30–90 sec	High
Strength	>85%	6–10	2–6	2–5 min	Medium
Power	>90%	1–5	3–5	~5 min	Low

Quick Reference: Determining Strength Training Experience[112]

Experience Level	Are they working out?	Length of training	Days per week to lift	Intensity of program
Beginner	No /just started	<2 months	< 1–2 days/wk	Very little
Moderate experience	Yes	2–6 months	<2–3 days/wk	Moderate
Experienced	Yes	> 1 year	>3–4 days/wk	High

Weight Lifting Belts

When people get their first weight set, they usually purchase a weightlifting belt, too. However, are they needed? In theory, weightlifting belts help by increasing the pressure inside of the abdominal cavity (intra-abdominal pressure) to help stabilize the lower core muscles and the spinal cord, which in theory reduces low back injuries. Some lifters also feel that belts increase lifting performance.[128] Studies, however, note that many people use belts for the wrong reasons.[128] Many experts recommend that weightlifting belts only be used for maximal or near maximal lifts that stress the low back.[78] Trainers should also remember that studies on weightlifting belts have not consistently found that they improve performance or reduce injury risk.[128] One possible negative side effect of using belts on a regular basis is that they may weaken the back muscles as the body grows accustomed to the help that belts provide. Moreover, people who experience pain during lifts should not rely on a belt. Pain is a signal that something is wrong. In this case, the pain-eliciting exercise should be halted and the lifter referred to his or her physician, who can make the appropriate diagnosis.

Periodization

Ultimately, periodization is what we have been reviewing in this chapter up to this point. Periodization refers to breaking up workouts into different **periods** or cycles. During each cycle, the weight, repetitions, sets, exercise selection, rest periods, and exercise order are specifically chosen to help reduce injury and improve fitness levels. At the start of the program, stress is kept low and not specific to any body part or goal. As fitness improves, the stress of the workout is increased and becomes more focused on the person's goals or needs.

Central to periodization is the notion of how the body adapts to stressors applied to it. The body adapts to any form of stress in stages. The process that describes these stages is referred to as the **General Adaptation Syndrome** (GAS), first proposed by scientist Hans Selye. According to GAS, the body goes through three phases as it adapts. The **alarm phase** is the first stage. Here, the person tends to experience DOMS and muscle stiffness as the body tries to cope with the stress of a new exercise program. Exercise performance may fluctuate for several weeks during this stage as the body adapts. During the **resistance phase,** the body slowly begins to adapt to the exercise and begins to grow stronger due to muscular growth, biochemical changes, and various neurological alterations. If, however, the same stimulus is applied for too long or is increased too quickly, the body begins to break down and become weaker and more prone to injury. This is called the **exhaustion phase.** During the exhaustion phase, **overtraining syndrome** might occur. The trick is to keep people in the adaptation phase and to avoid the exhaustion phase at all costs. The best way to do this is by altering programs periodically, using periodization.

Generally, there are three major cycles in periodization. A **macrocycle** is the largest cycle and encompasses an entire year of training. Each macrocycle is made up of several **mesocycles,** which can last from weeks to several months. Each mesocycle, is then made up of many **microcycles,** which are about a week long. Remember, a person's fitness level, physical limitations, age, and time commitment will all dictate how long these cycles really last. For example, you could have microcycles lasting a month.

Within the cycles of periodization are several distinct parts called **periods** and **phases.** Let us review the periods and phases now, keeping in mind that while periodization was originally designed for "athletes," its principles can be applied to anyone. Athlete or not, the major goals of periodization are reduction in injury and boredom and optimal physical performance over time.

The **preparatory period** is usually taken to be the first stage of periodization and is where many people will focus the majority of their efforts. It is here that the preparation work is done to ready the person for his or her ultimate goal or competition. This period is composed of three distinct phases: hypertrophy phase, strength phase, and power phase.

In the **hypertrophy phase,** to goal is to provide a foundation of muscular hypertrophy and endurance. Notice that *endurance* is part of this phase. Untrained muscles usually have little endurance. During this phase, the sets can be anywhere from 2–3, depending on fitness level. The loads are generally light or moderate and the number of repetitions is somewhat higher (12–20). Depending on fitness level, age, and health issues, the sets, repetitions, and resistances used may be less than this. For beginners, it is not always necessary to determine exact strength values (e.g., 10RM). Doing so may expose people to injury or DOMS. It is important to avoid overwhelming them while still challenging them enough to fatigue the muscles within 12–20 repetitions. The intensity during this phase is generally low, while volume of exercise (weight x repetitions x sets) is medium to high. While workouts usually occur 2–3 times a week, use your good judgment when deciding this. This phase may last up to 8 weeks and can even go longer if you deem it necessary.

During the **strength phase,** the intensity of the workout is increased. For healthy people, it generally entails 2–6 sets of 4–10 repetitions performed at about 85% 1RM, 2–4 days a week. For many people, periodization can stop here (or at the hypertrophy phase). Once a person reaches his or her desired level of strength, endurance, or hypertrophy, it is not always necessary to progress to the power phase.

During the **power phase,** the intensity of workouts increases and exercises become more specific to what the person's goals are. Also, the volume of the workouts decreases accordingly. This is done to avoid injury and, in the case of athletes, to prevent him or her from feeling overwhelmed as competition approaches.

Usually, the power phase requires performing 3–5 sets of 1–5 repetitions at an intensity of 75–95% of the 1RM.[78] Because some ADLs may require muscular power (e.g., crossing a busy street), the trainer needs to use his or her good judgment regarding whether to include this phase in a training program. When working with non-athletes, examine the person's goals, ADLs, injuries, age, and other limitations before attempting the power phase.

Following the power phase, some trainers may include a brief active rest period, often called the **first transition period,** to give the person a break from the rigors of tough training. This may last for a week or two. After this, comes the **competition period**. With respect to athletes, the competition period is the time during which they are actively participating in their sport. The focus here is not necessarily on exhaustive workouts, but rather on more specific sports-oriented tasks. During this time, the intensity of exercise is high (i.e., >90% 1RM) while volume is low, with around 3_5 sets of 1_5 repetitions performed. For non-athletes, the competition phase is usually not needed.

Following the competition period is a time of active rest called the **second transition period,** in which the person takes a break from intense training and participates in recreational activities for 1– 4 weeks.[78] After this, goals can be reassessed and another macrocycle can be planned for the following year.

Is this all that there is to periodization? No—periodization is a complex topic and there are many good books available to help those who want to learn more. See www.Joe-Cannon.com/Resources for a list of resources that I recommend. The goal here was to provide a foundation upon which to build.

It is important to remember that periodization is really a fluid concept rather than one that is fixed and unyielding. As such, the rules given here for sets, repetition schemes, and weight are generally textbook guidelines and should not be taken as "gospel" for all people. Fitness trainers are more likely to encounter untrained novices than athletes. Thus, age, desire to train, health issues, and goals can all impact how quickly one progresses. While most clients may not progress as quickly as the outlines here suggest, periodization can still help all people achieve greater results over time. If your first rules of thumb are "do no harm" and "progress people slowly," periodization can be a great benefit to your clients and will separate you from others who do not use this powerful training tool.

Periodization Quick Reference

Period/Phase	Details/Goals
Preparatory Period	Builds foundation for future training.
Hypertrophy Phase	Muscular hypertrophy and muscular endurance. High volume, low resistances.
Strength Phase	Increase strength. Intensity increases, volume decreases.
Power Phase*	Develop explosive strength. Intensity increases, volume decreases.
Competition Period*	High intensity, low volume. Sports-specific movements.
Active Rest (Transition) Period	Recreational activities. Gives body time to recuperate.

* May not be needed in non-athletes

Types of Strength Programs

There are many different types of strength training programs. This section reviews some of the most commonly used types. Keep in mind that variations of each program exist and research does not generally find one system to be better than another for all people. All programs have their place and their limitations. The key for the exercise professional is to decide which program balances safety, effectiveness, and appropriateness for the person with whom he or she is working.

Single-Set Programs: Single-set programs typically work the total body in a session and are some of the easiest to design. They usually consist of performing only one set of an exercise per body part. For example, one might do a chest press, followed by a lat pull down, followed by a leg press. After completing one exercise for each of the major muscle groups, the person is finished. The resistance used is generally heavy enough to fatigue the muscle within about 12–20 repetitions. Single-set programs share some things in common with circuit training but generally do not incorporate a cardiovascular component. Cardio can be performed separately, either before or after the program, or on an alternate day depending on time, goals, fatigue level, and health profile.

Circuit Training: This mode of strength training is a total body program that requires the lifter to use lighter resistances and to move from one exercise to another with little or no rest in between. If rest periods are used, they are kept short, usually fewer than 30 seconds. Generally, 8–15 exercises targeting the major muscle groups make up a circuit, but this may vary considerably. A well-designed circuit ensures that no single muscle group receives too much stress. If one completes the circuit and has enough time and energy, the circuit can be performed again.

While machines are typically used in circuits, free weight circuits or circuits using both machines and free weights can be used. Stability balls, elastic tubing, calisthenics, and other tools can also be used. The design of an exercise circuit is limited only by one's imagination. Many "boot camps" have their origins in circuit training. While typically considered to improve only strength, circuits also can improve power, flexibility, and aerobic capacity. Some research suggests that circuit training can improve aerobic capacity by about 4% in men and about 8% in women over the course of 20 weeks of training.[142] Other research has noted that aerobic capacity may improve by up to 51%.[143] For added benefit and variety, treadmills, bikes, and other pieces of cardiovascular equipment can also be added to the exercise circuit.

Besides being fun and not boring, circuit training offers a reduced risk of injury relative to other strength training programs, making it a very attractive option for beginners. Another major benefit is that circuits are usually deemed as the safest type of workout regimen for those with a number of medical issues ranging from heart disease to hypertension, cancer, and arthritis, to name a few.[141] Circuit training also lends itself well to those with limited time to exercise and can be made quite challenging if designed appropriately.

Isometric Programs: Isometric programs involve pressing or pulling against immovable objects. For example, pressing the hands together on front of the chest is an isometric chest exercise. Another name for this is "static contractions," a name given because no sliding of actin and myosin occurs during the activity. Probably the most famous isometric exercise is the "plank." Isometrics may be employed in some physical therapy settings to help deconditioned or injured individuals. In therapy, however, they are almost certainly progressed to more challenging (isotonic) movements eventually.

Isometric exercise can improve strength and power, but this appears for the most part to be limited to the joint angle used during the movement. Some research also hints that longer recovery periods between sets may be required when performing isometric movements.[181] Also, some studies suggest that isometrics may increase blood pressure more than traditional resistance training programs, making isometrics inappropriate for some with heart disease and/or high blood pressure, especially when combined with the Valsalva maneuver.

Multiple-Set Programs: Multiple-set programs entail performing more than one set of an exercise. For example, a person might do 3 sets of 10 repetitions of a bench press. Rest periods lasting anywhere from fewer than 30 seconds to 5 minutes are typically used between sets, depending on the training goal. Within the multiple-set arena, variations are possible and might include such as keeping the load constant and increasing or decreasing the load on subsequent sets (e.g., pyramid sets).

So, what is better for strength—one set or multiple sets? Even in beginners, research finds that multiple sets can produce greater strength than single-set programs.[144] That said, in novices, multiple sets will cause more DOMS, which may result in a greater drop-out rate. Also, doing multiple sets with beginners or with people who have health issues may put the individual at greater risk of injury. Another consideration is that, while multiple sets may develop more strength, the difference in strength gained in single-set programs is often not significantly less in the beginning.[144] Because of this, along with the increased time commitment and possible increase in injury, single-set programs may be best or safest for the first couple of months of training. Beyond this point, though, multiple sets are superior.

Split-Routine Programs: Split routines refer to any program that splits training into separate days. Each day, a different body part or group of body parts is emphasized. The advantage of a split routine is that one can focus more heavily on individual muscle groups. For example, one might spend a day working just chest and biceps.

Because split routines allow for greater intensity yet do not require a person to spend hours in the gym; they are quite popular with bodybuilders and athletes. Split routines also allow more rest between workouts. The downside is that split routines typically require spending more days in the gym, which may not be ideal for beginners. Technically, one could work out 7 days in a row if he or she really wanted to.

While popular among advanced lifters, the little research that exists hints that split routines may not be the best way for novices to train. For example, one study looked at 5 months of training with either a whole body program or a split routine in 30 untrained young women.[146] In spite of the differences in routines, similar results were obtained.

Superset Programs: When someone does a superset, he or she may be performing one of two separate but similar types of programs. One type of supersetting involves performing two exercises back-to-back that target opposing muscle groups. For example, one might perform a leg extension followed by a leg curl. Typically, little or no rest is taken between the exercises. By targeting opposing muscle groups, one muscle rests while the other is working.

Another type of supersetting involves performing 2 or 3 different exercises for the *same* muscle group with little rest. For example, one might do a set of dumbbell biceps curls followed by a set of spider curls. Supersetting is popular with advanced lifters and with those who have limited time to work out.

Push/Pull Programs: In a push/pull program, the lifter generally performs all of the pushing exercises (bench press, leg press, etc.) on one day followed by all the pulling movements (lat pull down, biceps curl, etc.) on another day. Thus, push/pull programs can be considered a type of split routine. A variation of this program is to perform a pushing movement followed immediately by a pulling exercise. In this respect, push/pull programs are very similar to supersetting. One advantage of push/pull programs is that they are time efficient, allowing multiple sets to be performed in a limited amount of time. They are also very aggressive, so they may be difficult for novices to perform.

Pyramid Programs: With pyramid programs, the lifter usually begins with a light resistance that he or she can lift for about 10–12 repetitions. In subsequent sets, the lifter increases the weight by 2.5–10 pounds, which results in a decrease in the number of repetitions that can be performed. Eventually, the lifter reaches the "top of the pyramid" and can only perform one or a few repetitions. After this point, the weight is reduced by 2.5–10 pounds, resulting in more repetitions being able to be performed. At the "bottom of the pyramid," the lifter is once again back to his or her starting point.

A variation of the pyramid program requires the lifter to perform only half of the pyramid. This is frequently referred to as "up pyramiding" (or ascending pyramiding) and "down pyramiding" (or descending pyramiding). An up pyramid is begins with the trainee using a light resistance and gradually increasing the resistance. A down pyramid begins with the client using a heavy resistance and reducing the weight on subsequent lifts.

So, which type of pyramid program is better? Little research proves conclusively the superiority of one system over another. Both have their place in a strength training program, and periodically alternating between systems may produce better results than either program alone. For beginners, though, performing either system is likely to be difficult, may result in DOMS, and, in theory, may increase one's risk for injury.

Eccentric-Only Training Programs: This type of program consists of only performing eccentric muscle actions, also called "negatives." While greater force production does appear to occur during eccentric muscle actions, interestingly, studies that directly compare concentric-only muscle actions to eccentric-only muscle actions are mixed, with some finding that eccentrics are better and others finding no difference.[77, 147] Other research suggests that eccentric-only repetitions may be superior for the development of muscle hypertrophy.[148] Still other research finds that performing a heavy eccentric repetition just prior to performing a concentric repetition enhances the lifter's 1RM.[151]

For those who wish to try this mode of training, there are several options. Some computerized strength machines allow the lifter to enter a light resistance during the concentric phase and a very heavy resistance during the eccentric phase. It is also possible to perform eccentric-only repetitions by using a lifting partner or, if using a selectorized machine, by lifting the heavy weight with both limbs and lowering it with only one limb (for example, during a leg extension). Lifting partners might also apply additional manual resistance during the eccentric phase.

Regardless of how you look at it, performing only eccentric repetitions is an advanced form of strength training that may result in injury if used with beginners. Eccentric muscle actions also increased the risk for rhabdomyolysis, a very serious medical disorder. In my opinion, this type of training should not be performed unless the lifter has been consistently involved in heavy strength training for at least one year.

Super Slow Programs: In super slow programs, the weight is lifted very slowly. One popular method calls for 10 seconds to be spent lifting the weight and 5 seconds to be spent lowering the weight.[149] Some research suggests that super slow training may augment strength in untrained individuals.[150] Other research suggests that super slow exercises may not be optimal for weight loss in experienced lifters because fewer calories are generally used.[149.] Conversely, by forcing the individual to perform the exercise slowly, super slow programs may lead to fewer injuries. They may therefore lend themselves well to those trying to work around current injuries.

Interval Training Programs: Interval training, also called High Intensity Interval Training (HITT), is a program in which people alternate the exercise intensity during a workout. There are periods of high intensity (the work period) followed by a period of low intensity (the recovery period) with a short period of time (for example, about 1 minute) in between. In this way, HITT is somewhat analogous to super sets.

Research finds that interval training can improve both aerobic and anaerobic fitness as well as the size and number of mitochondria. EPOC has also been shown to increase in interval training. Because interval training involves bursts of high intensity activity, yields many of the same benefits as traditional steady-state exercise in a shorter amount of time. This and other advantages have made HITT popular with fitness trainers.

While HITT has many benefits, steady state exercise (e.g., walking for 30 minutes) is likely the safest option for novices when they begin training. One reason for this is that beginners may lack the coordination to move at faster speeds. Also, as intensity increases (around 55% Karvonen HR), greater levels of hydrogen ions (lactic acid) are produced. This could result in vomiting in those not accustomed to HITT. In beginners, HITT will also cause DOMS. Moreover, for those with medical issues, HITT may need to be modified or replaced with less aggressive forms of activity. Also, because novices cannot complete high-volume workouts at first, the number of calories used during HITT is lower than the number burned during lower intensity, longer lasting steady-state exercise.

It is wise to remember that HITT does not have to appear the same for every individual. The idea—especially for novices—is to get people a little bit beyond their comfort zone for a short time. This could be accomplished with something as simple as walking a bit faster than normal for 20–30 seconds.

When discussing interval training with clients, it may be wise to refrain from calling it "HITT," as this term gives the impression that all benefits are tied to the "high intensity" portion. Cardiovascular adaptations also occur during the recovery period. Theoretically, workouts that consist solely of high intensity exercises could take the "interval" out of interval training. For teaching purposes, a better name for this program might be "high/low training" because this phrase places the emphasis on both aspects.

It is best to introduce HITT slowly. For example, after a month or two of steady-state exercise, begin with only 1 "round" (1 high-intensity period and 1 recovery period) per session for the first week. Perform 2 "rounds" in the second week, and so on. Also, to be extra safe, make the rest period 2–3 times longer than the work period at first. For example, if someone runs for 1 minute, have them walk for 2–3 minutes afterward. As fitness improves, the rest period can be decreased.

Tips for Interval Training

Warm up first for about 5 minutes	Remember that "high intensity" does always have to be overwhelming to the person
Cool down for about 5 minutes afterwards	Make recovery period 2–3 times longer than work period at first
RPE scale is usually better than HR	Introduce HITT slowly
Do not overlook the rest period	Build an aerobic fitness foundation with steady state exercise before starting HITT
To improve, increase either the intensity (number of repetitions) or the time of the program—but not both at the same time	Consider the client's health issues

Chapter 9

EXERCISE TECHNIQUE

This chapter deals with the proper way to perform a variety of strength training exercises. Each exercise is broken down according to the major muscles used, spotting tips, and various comments and suggestions regarding the exercise in question. To facilitate learning, movements are also broken down into their concentric and eccentric phases. While there are hundreds of different types of strength training activities, this chapter will deal with 50 of the most common (and some not-so-common) exercises with which fitness trainers should be familiar.

SEATED MACHINE CHEST PRESS

Primary Muscles Worked: Pectoralis major, anterior deltoids, triceps.

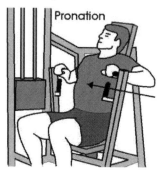

Quick Tip: The neutral grip is usually easier on the shoulders than the pronated grip shown here.

Exercise Technique: Adjust the seat height so that the handles are about parallel with the nipple line of chest. Usually, the feet are on the floor or floor plate of the machine with the thighs parallel to the floor. Grasp the handgrips, keeping the forearms parallel to the floor. Wrists should not be bent. Wrap the thumbs around handgrips. The starting point is when the elbows are in line with the shoulders. The elbows should not be behind the torso. If lifting a heavy weight, pull the shoulder blades together (i.e., retract scapula) and try to maintain this retraction for the duration of the exercise. With lighter weights, pulling the shoulder blades together may not be needed.

Concentric phase: Slowly press forward and stop just before the elbows lock out (i.e., a "soft lockout"). Hold for 1 second.

Eccentric phase: Slowly lower weight to the starting position. However, do not let elbows travel past the point of the torso (or midline of the body).

Spotting: Wrists should be firm and straight and not bent. Thumbs should be wrapped around the handgrips. The fitness professional can stand in front of the machine, making sure that the lifter's form is correct, or stand behind or to the side of the machine. Standing behind or to the side may be easier to cue the person regarding when to halt the eccentric phase of the exercise.

Comments & Suggestions: The machine chest press is a multi-joint exercise designed to mimic the free weight bench press. Many chest press machines have two handgrip positions. The picture depicted here shows the more traditional, pronated position with the palms facing down. People with shoulder injuries may find the neutral position (with palms facing each other) easier on the shoulders. Some machines have a pedal or bar close to the floor against which the feet can press to bring the handles to a safe position for starting the exercise. This negates the need to reach back and bring the elbows past the torso, which can exacerbate shoulder injuries. On some versions of this machine, it is possible to maintain contact between the feet and the bar or pedal. Doing so may stop the handles from traveling back too far, saving the shoulders from potential harm. This can also teach beginners the correct ROM for the exercise.

The normal convention is to exhale when lifting the weight and inhale during the lowering phase. Novices may have trouble coordinating breathing and lifting. If this happens, instruct the person to count or talk during the lift. The end result is the same—maintaining proper blood pressure and avoiding the Valsalva maneuver.

BARBELL BENCH PRESS

Primary Muscles Worked: Pectoralis major and minor, anterior deltoids, triceps, serratus anterior.

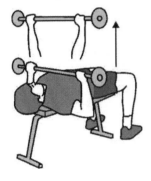

> **Quick Tip:** Retract the shoulder blades prior to performing this exercise with heavy resistances.

Exercise Technique: The barbell should have equal weight on both sides and be secured by collars. Adjust the height of the barbell such that there is a slight bend in the elbows when you grasp the barbell in the supine position. When supine on the bench, the barbell should be lined up with the eyes. The rest of the body should be evenly distributed on the bench with the feet on the floor at least shoulder-width apart, if not a little wider. Feet can be under the knees or a little in front of them. The spine should be neutral and not hyper-extended. Grasp barbell with a pronated grip, wrapping the thumbs around the bar. The wrists are straight and not bent. The grip should be about shoulder-width apart or a little wider. Hands and elbows are in line with each other. Begin by lifting the barbell off of its suspension hooks to a position in line with the chest. Arms are straight but elbows are not fully locked.

Eccentric phase: Lower the bar slowly, stopping when the elbow is at the level of the shoulder. At the end of the eccentric phase, the forearms should be perpendicular to the ground (in other words, there should be a 90° bend in arms). Do not bounce the barbell off of the chest. Pause for 1 second.

Concentric phase: Slowly press the barbell upward and stop just before the elbows are locked. Repeat for the desired number of repetitions.

Spotting: It is common for the trainer to stand behind the head of the lifter during this exercise. The trainer who spots this exercise usually will be in the "athletic position" (with abs tight and knees slightly bent). Trainers usually ask if the lifter needs a "lift off," or help getting the barbell off of the hooks and into its proper location over the chest. If the lifter answers yes, spotters often use an **alternated grip** (one hand supinated and the other pronated). The same grip is used at the end of the set if helping re-rack the barbell. Spotting is more than just helping with the lift off—it also involves identifying errors in lifting technique, giving verbal feedback and encouragement, and watching for signs that the lifter may be in danger (e.g., wobbling or unstable bar, shaking arms, arching back, or holding breath). At some point during the concentric phase, the lifter may reach his or her sticking point, or the most difficult point of the exercise, and may need help from the spotter during this time. Spotters should always ask the lifter how many repetitions he or she can perform so that they have a sense for when the lifter may need help. Remove weight plates from the barbell evenly. Taking too much weight off of only one side of the barbell may cause the barbell to flip over and cause injury.

Comments & Suggestions: The technique described above is commonly used by many people, but in some cases, this may result in rotator cuff shoulder injury. Thus, a narrower grip is sometimes advocated.[136] For most people, it is not necessary to touch the bar to the chest, as doing so might cause or exacerbate shoulder injuries. One way to teach a person how far to descend is to place a rolled up towel on the lifter's chest. When used, the elbows are usually in line with the shoulder when the bar contacts with the towel. Those involved in Olympic and Powerlifter's, though, train differently and need to adhere to the rules of their sports.

When calculating weight lifted, remember to count the Olympic bar (45 pounds) and the collars. One difference between barbells and dumbbells is that, because the barbell is a single weight, it is easier to balance than dumbbells. As such, people generally can lift more weight with barbells. Thus, it may be prudent to start with barbells and progress to dumbbells.

The lifter should keep his or her head on the bench at all times. Some research suggests that lifting the head off of the bench decreases the weight that can be lifted.[137] Strength trainers who lift heavy weights should be aware of a condition called **effort thrombosis**, in which blood clots form due to repeated trauma of the axillosubclavian vein in the upper body.[172] While rare, this condition may be more frequent in bodybuilders and heavy strength trainers. Signs can include pain and swelling in the neck and shoulders coupled with limited mobility. This condition requires immediate medical attention.

Common Bench Press Mistakes

Error	Reason
Bouncing barbell off chest	Barbell might crack sternum or cause other injury. It also means lifter did not take advantage of strength-enhancing eccentric phase of the exercise.
Lifting too much weight	Golgi tendon organ (GTO) relaxes muscles if it detects an injury. This will happen if too much weight is lifted.
Lifting too quickly	Places excessive stress on joints, increasing injury risk.
Arching the low back	Places excessive stress on low back muscles and spinal cord.
Not wrapping thumbs around bar	Barbell might roll out of hands.
Bending wrists	Places excessive force on delicate wrist bones.
Raising head off of bench	Stresses cervical neck area. May cause neck injury.
Shoulders arching to earlobes (seated chest press only)	Incorrect technique. May signify shoulders performing more work than they should.
Holding breath	Also known as "Valsalva maneuver." Might increase BP to dangerous levels.
Grip too wide	The wider the grip, the more stress on the shoulders.
Locking out elbows	May increase risk of injury to elbow joint.

DUMBBELL BENCH PRESS

Primary Muscles Worked: Pectoralis major and minor, anterior deltoids, triceps, serratus anterior.

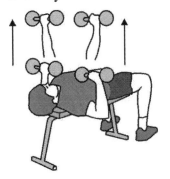

Quick Tip: During the eccentric phase, stop when the elbows are at or just a little below the torso.

Exercise Technique: Grasp two dumbbells of equal weight and sit on a stable exercise bench with dumbbells resting on your thighs. If necessary, perform hip flexion to use the thighs to help lift the dumbbells to shoulder level prior to lying supine on the bench. Lie supine on the bench with feet on the floor at least shoulder-width apart, if not wider. Head, shoulders, and buttocks should be evenly distributed on the bench. Wrists should be straight, not bent. The dumbbells should be at chest level and aligned with the nipple line. At all times during the exercise, keep the thumbs wrapped around the dumbbells. Rotate arms such that the elbows are pointed away from the body (i.e., are lateral to the torso). The elbows should be at the level of the shoulders. The forearms should be perpendicular to the floor and elbows in line with the shoulders.

Concentric phase: Slowly press dumbbells upward. Do not allow the dumbbells to sway back and forth or lose control of them at any point during the ROM. Press until soft lockout is reached. Do not arch the low back or remove the feet from the floor during the lift.

Eccentric phase: Slowly lower the dumbbells to the starting point and repeat for the desired number of repetitions. At the end of the exercise at the bottom of the last eccentric phase, rotate the elbows inward toward the body, sit up slowly, and rest the dumbbells on the thighs.

Spotting: It is common for trainers to be positioned behind the person's head and low to the ground during this exercise. During the eccentric phase, trainers may place their hands at the height of the shoulders to cue the lifter not to lower his or her elbows past this point. During the concentric phase, trainers may grasp the wrists of the client to help him or her steady the dumbbells and reduce risk of injury. Do not pull the dumbbells up by the wrists of the lifter, as this may result in shoulder injury, especially if the lifter is not expecting it. Ask the lifter how he or she wants to be spotted ahead of time. With very heavy dumbbells, it may be necessary to hand the lifter the dumbbells prior to performing the exercise. If this occurs, the spotter should *not* hold the dumbbell by the handgrip. Doing so prevents the lifter from grasping the dumbbell safely. Rather, grasp each end of the dumbbell and hand dumbbells to the lifter on at a time.

Comments & Suggestions: It is important to maintain a closed grip on dumbbells at all times during the exercise. Failure to do so may lead to injury. Note the height of the bench. A bench that is too high may cause one to arch the lower back. If this happens, have the trainee place the feet on a raised platform or an aerobic step to alleviate the problem. Placing the feet on the bench is also an option, but remember that when the feet are on the bench, the lifter's base of support narrows, which might lead to falling off the bench.

The dumbbells do not have to clank together at the top of the lift. Doing so may cause the paint of some dumbbells to flake off and get in the individual's eyes. Depending on shoulder stability and pain-free ROM, the dumbbells can be kept in the same plane of motion or moved closer together during the concentric phase. Lifters sometimes lower the dumbbells to points at which the elbows are far below the torso because they want to "feel the stretch." However, this practice removes stress from the chest muscles and places more stress on the shoulder joint—one of the weakest areas of the body. This is why one does not have to lower dumbbells past the torso line for this exercise to be effective. This exercise can also be performed using a neutral grip, where the elbows are closer to the body and palms face each other. This grip generally places less stress on the shoulder. Some people may, at the end of the lift, simply drop the weights on the floor while they are supine on the bench. This can lead to shoulder injury. In addition, anyone nearby may be injured. Thus, this practice should be avoided.

PUSH-UPS ON THE STABILITY BALL

Primary Muscles Used: Pectoralis major, anterior deltoids, triceps, serratus anterior, posterior deltoids, rectus abdominis, core musculature.

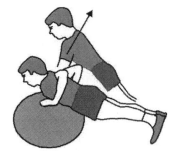

Quick Tip: Be proficient at regular push-ups before attempting. Placing the feet closer together increases the difficulty of this exercise.

Exercise Technique: Obtain a properly inflated stability ball and place the hands on the top outer and upper sides of the ball, about shoulder-width apart, with fingers oriented downward toward the sides of the ball. In this position, the elbows will be closer to the body and not flared out at the sides. The legs are extended and are shoulder-width apart or wider, with the bodyweight on the toes.

Eccentric phase: Slowly lower the upper torso down to the ball while keeping the ball in line with the chest. Halt the movement when the elbows are at the level of the torso or when comfortable.

Concentric phase: Press down on the ball, lifting the torso to starting point, while again keeping the ball in line with the chest. Stop just before the elbows lock out. Hold position for a second or two. Repeat.

Spotting: The low back should not slouch downward. The head should stay neutral, neither lifting up nor turning to the sides. The hands may slide off the ball if sweaty.

Comments & Suggestions: This is an advanced form of push-ups that challenges the entire core musculature and requires considerable strength and endurance. This can also be an effective shoulder stabilizing exercise for overall shoulder health. This movement requires considerable core strength. The core is sometimes mentioned in relation to the abs and low back muscles, but it really includes all of the muscles in the trunk. The gluteals, for example, are part of the core.

Another version of this exercise is to perform the push-up with hands on the floor and ankles resting on the ball. One limiting factor to performing this movement may be the extreme pressure placed on the wrists. While it may seem that this exercise would be easier with an under-inflated ball, this is not so.

DUMBBELL FLY

Primary Muscles Worked: Pectoralis major, anterior deltoid

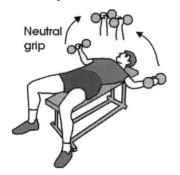

Neutral grip

Quick Tip: Halt the eccentric phase when the elbows are at the level of the shoulders.

Exercise Technique: Obtain two dumbbells of equal weight and lay supine on a stable exercise bench. Use a closed grip for the duration of the exercise. Wrists are rigid and not bent during the exercise. Extend arms to a soft lockout position (slight bend in elbows) with a neutral grip (palms facing each other). The arms should be at or just below shoulder level. In this position, the elbows should be pointed outward, away from the body.

Eccentric phase: Slowly lower the arms while maintaining a soft lockout in the elbows. Traditionally, the eccentric phase stops when the elbows are at or slightly above the shoulder line (or the midline of the body), although individual biomechanics will dictate the safe ROM.

Concentric phase: Raise the arms back to the starting point using a "hugging motion." Elbows remain in soft lockout throughout the exercise. Repeat for the desired number of repetitions.

Spotting: It is important that both the lifter and spotter agree ahead of time on how the dumbbells will be handled off at the end of the lift. Will the spotter take them from the lifter's hands, or will the lifter rise up and rest them on his or her thighs? Proper communication between the lifter and spotter can reduce risk of injury during this critical period of the exercise.

During this exercise, the spotter is positioned behind the lifter's head while kneeling on one or two knees. The spotter watches the plane of motion of the dumbbells, the lifter's expression, and other body cues. During the concentric phase of the lift, the spotter keeps his or her hands near the lifter's wrists. It is not necessary to grasp the wrists unless the lifter is in imminent danger of dropping the weights. During the eccentric phase, the spotter also keeps his or her hands close to the lifter's wrists and may alternate by placing the hands at shoulder level to signal to the lifter to avoid lowering the weight past this point.

Comments & Suggestions: One common error with this exercise is trying to press the weights as if performing a bench press. Another error is over-accentuating elbow flexion. In general, the elbows should not be bent more than about 15–20°.

Some research shows that dumbbell flys may not be as effective at strengthening the pectoralis major and anterior deltoids as barbell or dumbbell bench presses.[129] The dumbbell fly is controversial in some circles in that it may contribute to rotator cuff shoulder injury or exacerbate existing rotator cuff issues. This can occur in many exercises in which the arm is abducted from the midline of the body or the elbows travel past shoulder level. Therefore, this exercise is probably best used with lighter weights. While the machine version is safest, it should also be reserved for those without shoulder problems.

PEC DECK (MACHINE PEC FLY)

Primary Muscles worked: Pectoralis major, anterior deltoid

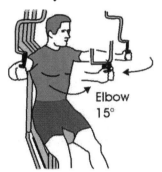

Elbow
15°

> **Quick Tip:** Some versions double as a reverse fly machine. In this case, ensure the handles are properly oriented before using.

Exercise Technique: Adjust the movable arms of the machine so that they are in line with the chest (or a little in front of it) when the individual sits in the machine. Sit facing away from the machine. The seat should be adjusted so that the handles are aligned with the nipple line of the chest. Grasp the handles with a closed grip. The elbows should be slightly bent. Wrists should be rigid and not hyper-flexed.

Concentric phase: Slowly bring the handles together in a controlled fashion, stopping just before the hands touch.

Eccentric phase: Slowly release to starting position and repeat.

Spotting: Trainers should ensure that the seat is at the proper height, that the elbows are slightly bent, and that the elbows do not travel behind the torso during the eccentric phase of the exercise.

Comments & Suggestions. Remind people that many machines of this type can double as a rear delt machine by simply altering the range of motion pins, which are usually located near the top of the device. People are often unaware of this, so when they try to use a pec deck that has been adjusted to work the rear delts, they have to reach extremely far back to grasp the handles, leading to shoulder injury as they perform the exercise with exaggerated ROMs. Also take this opportunity to remind people that greater ROM does not always mean greater chest development.

Some variations of this machine call for the lifter to place his or her forearms on pads. If this is the case, it is still important to ensure that the elbows do not travel past the torso.

REAR DELT MACHINE/REVERSE FLY

Primary Muscles Worked: Posterior deltoids, latissimus dorsi, rhomboids.

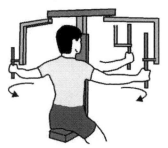

Quick Tip: Pull the shoulder blades together prior to starting this exercise.

Exercise Technique: If this is a piece of equipment that can double as a pec fly, adjust the machine to work the rear delts and sit facing the machine. The chest should be against the pad. Adjust the seat such that the handles are at chest height. Grasp handles and retract shoulder blades.

Concentric phase: While keeping a slight bend in the elbows, slowly bring the arms back and outward from the body. Stop when the elbows are in line with the shoulders.

Eccentric phase: Slowly return the arms to the starting position. Stop just before the weights touch the weight stack. Repeat for the desired number of repetitions.

Spotting: Make sure that the shoulder blades are retracted and that the elbows do not travel past the torso. The lifter's chest should not come off of the chest pad. Doing so is cheating and might indicate that the weight is too heavy. The lifter should not turn his or her head, but rather look straight ahead.

Comments & Suggestions: Since the rear deltoids are often used during lat pull downs, seated rows, and other back exercises, it is a personal decision whether to incorporate this exercise. Those performing this movement often force their arms as far back as possible, which may place too much stress on the shoulders. This exercise can also be performed with dumbbells or exercise tubing.

PRONE REVERSE FLY WITH STABILTY BALL

Primary Muscles Used: Posterior deltoids, latissimus dorsi, rhomboids, rotator cuff.

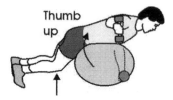

Thumb up

Quick Tip: This can also be performed on a bench if a stability ball is not available.

Exercise Technique: Obtain two light, equally weighted dumbbells and lay prone on a stability ball with the ball at the naval. The legs should be extended about hip- to shoulder-width apart with a slight bend at the knees. The head should be neutral and the abs contracted. The exercise is begun with the arms extended outward from the body (maintain a slight bend at the elbows) below the plane of the torso. The hands are oriented so that the thumbs are pointed up. In some variations, this is performed with the hands in the pronated position.

Concentric phase: Slowly raise the arms upward while keeping the shoulder blades pulled together. Stop when the arms are about shoulder height.

Eccentric phase: Slowly return arms to starting position. Repeat.

Spotting: The head stays neutral. The shoulder blades remain contracted. The trunk does not round forward over the ball.

Comments & Suggestions: This is a good rear deltoid exercise and goes well with external rotations and other movements designed to strengthen the rotator cuff. This exercise can also be performed without dumbbells. In such instances, the thumbs should point up toward the ceiling. An easier yet equally effective version of this exercise is performed with knees bent and on the floor.

LAT PULL DOWN

Primary Muscles Worked: Latissimus dorsi, posterior deltoid, rhomboids, teres major, trapezius.

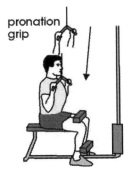

pronation grip

> **Quick Tip:** Pull the shoulder blades together prior to pulling the bar downward.

Exercise Technique: Sit facing the lat pull down machine and grasp the bar with an overhand grip. Hand placement on the bar will vary according to individual biomechanics and current or previous injuries, but in general, the hands remain about shoulder-width apart or a little wider. There should be a slight bend in the elbows and elbows should be pointed outward. Lean back slightly (15–45°). Retract the shoulder blades.

Concentric phase: Slowly pull the bar downward to the front of the head. Stop when the upper arms are about parallel with the floor. Hold for 1 second.

Eccentric phase: Slowly let the bar rise to the starting position and repeat. Do not let the bar go so high that the elbows lock out. Always maintain a slight bend in elbows. Repeat for the desired number of repetitions.

Spotting: The spotter stands behind the lifter and makes sure that the lifter is performing the exercise correctly. During heavy lifts, retract the shoulder blades. With lighter lifts, holding the retraction may not be needed. A good teaching cue for retraction is to have the person imagine having an ice cube dropped down his or her back. Alternatively, you may also place a finger between the trainee's shoulder blades and have them try to pinch your finger. Slightly leaning back (15–45°) is okay, but excessive lean is not. Likewise, rocking back and forth with each repetition is considered cheating and may increase risk of injury.

Comments & Suggestions: Pulling the bar behind the head is controversial because many believe that doing so may increase the risk of shoulder injury.[140] This movement may also strain the cervical neck or injure it if the bar impacts the neck during an overly forceful concentric phase. Some evidence suggests that pulling to the front of the head more effectively activates the lats than pulling behind the head.

With respect to hand placement, some research notes that an overhand grip actives the lats better than an underhand grip. Moreover, some advocate using a very wide grip to target the "outer lats." However, there is no such thing as "outer" or "inner" lats. Very wide grips may limit ROM and place greater stress on the shoulder joint, leading to injuries.

A variation of this exercise is to only retract the shoulder blades without pulling downward with the arms. Doing this works many of the same muscle groups and often allows more weight to be lifted.

SEATED ROW MACHINE

Primary Muscles Worked: Latissimus dorsi, rhomboids, trapezius, posterior deltoids.

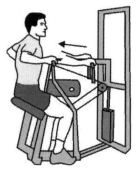

> **Quick Tip:** Retract shoulder blades prior to pulling with the arms.

Exercise Technique: Adjust the seat of the machine so that the chest is against the chest pad and the arms are about parallel to the floor when the individual is seated. If the machine has an adjustable chest pad, adjust it so that the lifter can reach the handles comfortably yet still have a slight bend in the elbows.

Concentric phase: Grasp handles with neutral grip. Retract shoulder blades and pull backward until the upper arm is about perpendicular to the floor. Hold for 1 second.

Eccentric phase: Slowly return to the starting position while maintaining shoulder retraction. Repeat for the desired number of repetitions.

Spotting: Stand behind the lifter and place your finger between his or her shoulder blades to prompt them into retraction. Have the trainee imagine what he or she would do if you suddenly dropped an ice cube down the back. Avoid rocking back and forth during the movement. If the shoulders roll forward, it is a sign that the weight may be too heavy.

Comments & Suggestions: On many pulling exercises, we advise lifters to retract their shoulder blades and hold the retraction throughout the movement. But is this always best? Generally, for heavier loads, this is ideal because it offers better trunk and shoulder stabilization. For lighter loads, though, holding the retraction may not be as important. In such situations, retracting and releasing the shoulder blades after each repetition merely offers variety to the exercise.

People may also perform this exercise on a seated pulley machine where the torso is not stabilized. If performed in this manner, rocking back and forth is not necessary and may strain the low back. Rather, the torso should remain in an upright posture throughout the exercise.

A variation of the seated row is to only retract the shoulder blades without pulling back with the arms. Doing this also works many of the same muscle groups and often allows for more weight to be lifted. It also is a good shoulder stabilizing exercise. The neutral grip is usually preferable to a pronated grip for those with shoulder injuries.

DUMBBELL ONE ARM BENT OVER ROW

Primary Muscles Worked: Posterior deltoids, latissimus dorsi, rhomboids, teres major.

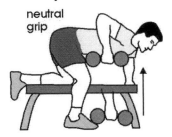
neutral grip

Quick Tip: Remember to retract the shoulder blade. The head should be neutral.

Exercise Technique: Obtain a dumbbell and place on the floor close to the front of a stable exercise bench. Place one knee on the exercise bench with the lower leg resting on the bench. The other foot remains on the floor pointed straight ahead with knee slightly bent. The hand that does not grasp the dumbbell is placed on the front or side of the exercise bench for stability. At this point, the trunk is about parallel with the bench. Body weight should be evenly distributed between the bent knee and hand. The head should be neutral, neither looking up nor to the sides. Grasp the dumbbell with a neutral grip. Abs should be contracted slightly.

Concentric phase: With the dumbbell in line with the shoulders, retract the shoulder blade and slowly pull the dumbbell upward until a 90° bend at the elbow is reached. At this point, the upper arm is parallel to the floor.

Eccentric phase: Slowly lower the dumbbell to the starting position while maintaining the retraction of the shoulder blades. Do not lock out the elbow at the bottom of the eccentric phase. The dumbbell should stay close to the body at all times. Repeat for the desired number of repetitions.

Spotting: People often twist the trunk in the direction of the pull in an attempt to help them lift the weight. This is cheating and is probably caused by lifting too much weight. Instead, the chest should remain facing down toward the floor. The head should stay neutral, neither looking upward nor to the sides.

Comments & Suggestions: While a flat bench is shown here, an adjustable bench elevated to about 30° can also be used. The knee and hand used for support should both be on the same side of the body. That is, if the left knee is bent, stabilize with the left hand and vice versa. For variety, this exercise can also be performed using an exercise ball, a selectorized machine, or with exercise tubing. This exercise may aggravate those with carpal tunnel syndrome because of the stress placed on the supporting hand.

MACHINE SHOULDER PRESS

Primary Muscles Worked: Anterior and medial deltoids, triceps, trapezius.

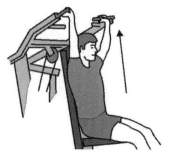

Quick Tip: Grasping the handles with palms facing each other reduces the stress on the shoulders.

Exercise Technique: In most versions of this exercise, the person sits facing away from the machine with the feet on the floor about hip width apart. The seat should be adjusted so that the thighs are about parallel with the floor. In the starting position, the elbows should be about shoulder height or a little lower. This may require reducing the seat height. The shoulders are weaker (due to less overlap between actin and myosin protein filaments) when the elbows are lower than shoulder height, which may limit the amount of weight that can be lifted. When the handles are grasped with a closed pronated grip, the elbows should point out from the sides of the body. The wrists are rigid and not bent backward.

Concentric phase: Press upward until soft lockout is reached.

Eccentric phase: Slowly lower until elbows are at shoulder height. Repeat for the desired number of repetitions.

Spotting: Common errors during this exercise include excessive arching of the low back, placing the hands too far apart (though this may be unavoidable with machines), turning the head during the lift, and not keeping the feet on the floor.

Comments & Suggestions: The shoulder press is sometimes considered controversial because few ADLs involve lifting heavy loads above the head. Use caution with this exercise if the lifter has any neck, shoulder, wrist, or elbow injuries. If the exercise is performed with a barbell, avoid pressing behind the head, as this may result in rotator cuff injuries. Many shoulder press machines allow this exercise to be performed with a neutral grip, which is usually considered safer for the shoulders.

LATERAL RAISE WITH DUMBELLS

Primary Muscles Worked: Medial deltoids.

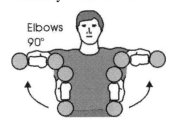

Elbows 90°

> **Quick Tip:** The elbows should go no higher than the shoulders.

Exercise Technique: Grasp two equally weighted dumbbells and stand with arms bent at 90°. The palms should be facing each other (neutral grip). If performed standing, the feet should be about hip- to shoulder-width apart. Lean slightly forward at the hips.

Concentric phase: Slowly raise the dumbbells until the elbows are at the height of the shoulders.

Eccentric phase: Slowly lower the dumbbells to the starting position.

Spotting: Make sure that the elbows do not travel higher than the shoulders, as this may increase one's risk of developing shoulder problems or exacerbate existing shoulder problems.

Comments & Suggestions: This exercise can be performed either seated or standing. Typically, this exercise is performed with arms extended outward from the sides of the body. If doing this version, remember to keep a slight bend in the elbows. The exercise shown here is a modified

105

version that takes stress off of the elbows. Because the shoulder is not very strong in this position, it is not necessary to use heavy weights.

Gyms typically have machines for this exercise. If using a machine, raise the seat height so that the shoulders are in line with the rotational points of the machine. On some machines, the rotational point is often highlighted by a colored plastic cover or sticker. Also, with machines, try not to grasp the handles too tightly, as this is cheating. Allow the shoulders to do the majority of the lifting.

This exercise may exacerbate rotator cuff injuries. A safer alternative to the lateral raise is **scaption,** whereby the lifter holds a light weight (or resistance band) with the arms at the sides but slightly forward (~30°) and thumbs pointing up. In this position, raise the nearly straightened arms (soft lockout at the elbow) until they are at about the height of the shoulders, then lower to the starting position.

The Rotator Cuff

Because of its great ROM, the shoulder is very prone to injury. One commonly injured are is the rotator cuff. The rotator cuff represents four muscles that keep the upper arm bone (the humerus) in its socket (the glenoid fossa) and is very active during all shoulder exercises. The muscles of the rotator cuff are the supraspinatus, infraspinatus, subscapularis and teres minor. Rotator cuff injuries are common in baseball, tennis, basketball, weightlifting, swimming, or any activity during which the arms are regularly raised over the head.

Common signs of rotator cuff injuries include shoulder pain, especially when reaching over the head, when lifting weights (e.g., bench pressing, doing push-ups, or performing a shoulder press), or when reaching the arm behind the back. Sometimes the pain occurs when not moving and may even cause an almost complete lack of mobility in the arm. In extreme cases, there may be a tear in the rotator cuff muscles, which may require surgery. Usual treatment includes ice to relieve inflammation, resting the muscle, and halting the activity that caused the injury. A physician may inject steroids (e.g., cortisone) into the area, prescribe pain relievers, and refer the person to a physical therapist who can recommend various exercises to help strengthen the rotator cuff. Adding rotator cuff exercises to your workout cannot only help prevent rotator cuff injuries themselves, but may also help reduce the risk of reoccurrence.

UPRIGHT ROW

Primary Muscles Worked: Anterior, medial and posterior deltoids, trapezius, serratus anterior, brachialis, brachioradialis, biceps.

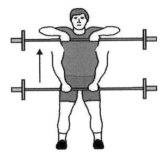

> **Quick Tip:** A wider grip may place less stress on the wrists and rotator cuff.

Exercise Technique: Stand erect and grasp an equally weighted barbell. The knees should be slightly flexed and the abs contracted with the hands pronated and closed around the barbell. Feet should be shoulder-width apart. The lifter should look straight ahead, with the back in a neutral position as opposed to "straight."

Concentric phase: Pull the bar slowly upward, keeping the bar close to the body at all times. Halt the exercise when the elbows are at the height of the shoulders. Avoid shrugging the shoulders during the exercise. Likewise, do not rise up on the toes.

Eccentric phase: Slowly lower the barbell until the arms are almost fully extended. Keep the bar close to the body at all times. Repeat for the desired number of repetitions.

Spotting: Make sure that the knees are slightly bent and that the elbows do not rise above shoulder height, as doing so may increase risk of shoulder injury. Ensure that the head does not turn to the sides.

Comments & Suggestions: The upright row is controversial in some circles in that it may increase the risk of shoulder injuries. As such, many trainers and physical therapists do not recommend it. During the concentric phase, the humorous may pinch the tendons of the rotator cuff, which may result in "impingement syndrome." As a general rule, the higher the elbows go, the greater the stress on the rotator cuff. As such, people with shoulder issues may want to avoid this exercise.

Traditionally, the upright row is performed with the hands held close together on the bar, which may place an excessive amount of force on the wrists. Some modify this exercise by using dumbbells or by holding the hands shoulder-width apart in the hopes of reducing the risk of shoulder and wrist injury. Another modification is to lift the elbows to shoulder height and no higher.

Controversial Exercises

Exercise	Reason
Upright rows	Possible increased risk of shoulder problems
Behind head military press	Possible increased risk of shoulder problems
Behind head lat pull down	Possible increased risk of shoulder problems
Good mornings	Possible increased risk of low back problems
Deep knee squats (>90°)	Possible increased risk of knee problems

EXTERNAL SHOULDER ROTATION WITH DUMBBELL

Primary Muscles Worked: Rotator cuff muscles (primarily infraspinatus and teres minor).

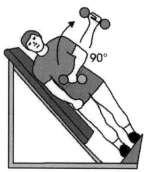

> **Quick Tip:** For added difficulty, perform on the floor.

Exercise Technique: Obtain a light dumbbell and lie on one's side on a stable incline exercise board (or the floor or a flat bench for added difficulty). The arm to be used should be bent at 90°. A towel can be placed beneath the head for comfort if desired.

Concentric phase: Rotate the bent arm outward from the body, stopping close to the end of the pain-free normal ROM or whenever the elbow moves away from the body.

Eccentric phase: Slowly lower to the starting position and repeat.

Spotting: A common error is moving the elbow away from the body. Having the lifter hold a towel between the elbow and torso should prevent this from occurring. Alternately, the spotter may place one or two fingers on the elbow to remind the lifter of the proper position.

Comments & Suggestions: People are usually stronger doing internal shoulder rotation than external rotation. Thus, an imbalance between these muscles might contribute to shoulder instability. For this reason, external shoulder rotation should be a staple in all exercise programs, especially since rotator cuff injuries are common in many sports. There are several variations of this exercise. For example, the exercise can be performed standing, using elastic tubing, or with no equipment if one uses his or her opposing hand to provide resistance. Normally, external and internal rotations are performed with lighter resistances and a higher number of repetitions (e.g., 15–20 repetitions).

SHOULDER FLEXION WITH DUMBBELLS

Primary Muscles Worked: Anterior deltoid, pectoralis major.

Neutral
grip

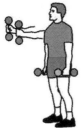

> **Quick Tip:** Performing with exercise tubing or a cable machine may strengthen the muscles over a greater ROM than dumbbells.

Exercise Technique: Obtain two equally weighted dumbbells and stand with feet shoulder-width apart with a slight bend in the knees and hips. The dumbbells should be held at the sides using a neutral grip. There should be a slight bend in the elbows at all times.

Concentric phase: Slowly raise the dumbbells up and in front of the body while maintaining a slight bend at the elbows. Stop when the hands are at about shoulder level (i.e., parallel with floor).

Eccentric phase: Slowly lower to the starting position. Repeat for the desired number of repetitions.

Spotting: The lifter should look straight ahead and not turn his or her head to the sides. The dumbbells should not tilt down at the wrists. If the wrists bend, this may signify that the weight is too heavy.

Comments & Suggestions: This exercise is also known as the front raise or front deltoid raise. Some people perform this exercise with a pronated (palms down) grip, which reduces the influence of the biceps muscles. Because the shoulder is relatively easy to injure and because this is a single joint exercise, work at higher numbers of repetitions (e.g., 15 repetitions) and keep the weight light. This exercise can also be performed seated, with exercise tubing, or using a cable machine.

Basic Shoulder Safety Guidelines

Warm up first	Stop if any sharp pain is felt
Maintain strength in rotator cuff	Use proper form
Avoid pressing behind the head	Do not lift more than you can safely handle
Avoid pulling the lat bar behind the head	Do not let elbows travel past the torso (e.g., during flys)

BARBELL SHRUG

Primary Muscles Worked: Upper trapezius, rhomboids, levator scapulae.

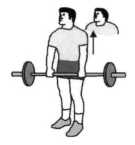

Quick Tip: Remember to keep a slight bend at the knees during this movement.

Exercise Technique: Hold an equally weighted barbell in front of the body. Alternatively, it can be held behind the body as well. Hands should be pronated and positioned a little wider than shoulder-width apart with the elbows slightly bent. There should also be a slight bend in the knees. The lifter will have a slight forward lean, which is okay.

Concentric phase: Slowly raise the shoulders upward. In this position, the shoulders will travel slightly behind the neck. This is okay.

Eccentric phase: Slowly lower the barbell to the starting point while maintaining a slight bend at the elbows. Repeat for the desired number of repetitions.

Spotting: The lifter's head should look straight ahead and not turn. There should be a small bend in the knees and the lifter should be slightly leaning forward to help efficiently recruit the appropriate muscles.

Comments & Suggestions: This exercise can also be performed with dumbbells, which can either be held at the sides or in front of the body. Regardless of which variation is used, it is not necessary to roll the shoulders while performing this exercise because doing so works the muscles perpendicular to gravity, which is an inefficient pattern of movement.

SUPINE LEG PRESS MACHINE

Primary Muscles Worked: Quadriceps (vastus lateralis, vastus medialis, vastus intermedius, rectus femoris), hamstrings (semimembranosus, semitendinosus, biceps femoris), gluteal muscles.

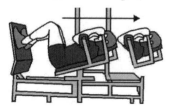

Quick Tip: Make sure toes are at least as high as knees.

Exercise Technique: Adjust the machine to the appropriate weight and recline with shoulders under the pads and feet on the metal platform. Feet should be hip-width apart with the toes at least as high as the knees if not a little higher.

Concentric phase: Press the feet into the foot plate, lifting the weight stack and halting just before a full knee lockout occurs.

Eccentric phase: Slowly lower the weight stack, halting just before the weights touch. Repeat for the desired number of repetitions.

Spotting: Ensure that the lifter's feet are at least as high as his or her knees and that the back is not arching. The spotter also reminds the lifter to breathe during the activity.

Comments & Suggestions: The supine leg press is one of several variations of this exercise. All basically challenge the same muscle groups similarly. Other popular types include the 45-degree leg sled and the seated leg press. One of the most common leg press mistakes is performing the exercise with the knees placed higher than (i.e., in front of) the toes. Doing so places **sheering forces** on the knees and can increase pain. Another common mistake is letting the knees bow inward during the lift. The knees should be at about hip- or shoulder-width apart during the lift. Arching of the low back may occur on the supine leg press when the lifter attempts to lift more weight than he or she can handle. If this occurs, it is prudent to reduce the resistance and lift the load more slowly. Some versions have a low back support to help reduce arching of the low back.

Leg Press vs. Squat

The leg press is often said to be a safer alternative to the squat performed with free weights. This point is debatable and really depends on the person in question. The squat is more sport-specific than the leg press. That is to say that athletics do not usually only involve leg strength but also require balance and strength of the entire core musculature. Because they tend to stabilize the low back and core, only performing leg presses might increase the risk of injury in athletes. One might make this point with the general population as well, given that many daily tasks require an integrated effort of the body rather than simply the legs. Conversely, it is generally easier to make lifting mistakes during a squat. Regardless, the real definition of which is safer depends on the person's unique health history and/or goals. For those with back injuries or balance issues, the leg press might be safer. Moreover, for novices, it is probably best to start by teaching the leg press and progress to the squat over time only if you deem it worthwhile.

SQUAT (WITH STABILITY BALL)

Primary Muscles Used: Quadriceps (vastus lateralis, vastus medialis, vastus intermedius, rectus femoris), hamstrings (semimembranosus, semitendinosus, biceps femoris), gluteal muscles, calves.

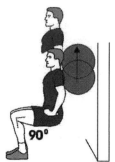

> **Quick Tip:** For added difficulty, use dumbbells and/or combine with biceps curl, lateral raise, or shoulder press.

Exercise Technique: Obtain a properly inflated stability ball and place it against a wall. Prior to the exercise, the ball should be positioned behind the lower back. Feet should be about shoulder-width apart with the toes pointing straight ahead. There should be a slight bend in the knees.

Eccentric phase: Slowly lower the body (as if sitting down in a chair), being mindful not to increase the lean of the torso during the descent and keeping the knees behind the toes. Descend to approximately 60° to 90° or to a comfortable level.

Concentric phase: Slowly rise up to the starting position, halting the movement just before knees lock out. Repeat for the desired number of repetitions.

Spotting: Ensure that the knees do not travel in front of the toes. If they do so, bring the feet further out from the wall and/or instruct the person to "push his or her buttocks into the wall."

Comments & Suggestions: Make sure that the person can do a wall squat and/or has sufficient balance before introducing the stability ball. For added difficulty, dumbbells, elastic tubing, or other forms of resistance may be used. Pressing through the heels places more stress on the glutes. If performing this exercise in the home, be aware that the ball may eventually leave a mark on the walls.

SQUAT (WITH DUMBBELLS)

Primary Muscles Used: Quadriceps (vastus lateralis, vastus medialis, vastus intermedius, rectus femoris), hamstrings (semimembranosus, semitendinosus, biceps femoris), gluteal muscles, calves.

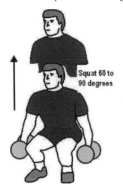

Squat 60 to 90 degrees

> **Quick Tip:** For added difficulty, perform while sitting down on a bench and/or rest dumbbells vertically on shoulders.

Exercise Technique: Obtain two equally weighted dumbbells and hold at the sides with a neutral grip. Feet should be about shoulder-width apart with the toes pointing straight ahead. There should be a slight bend in the knees.

Eccentric phase: Slowly lower the body (as if sitting down in a chair), being mindful not to let the knees travel past the toes. Descend to approximately 60° to 90° or to a comfortable level.

Concentric phase: Slowly rise up to the starting position, halting the movement just before the knees lock out. Repeat for the desired number of repetitions.

Spotting: Ensure that the knees do not travel beyond the toes when viewed from the side and that the heels do not come off of the floor during the exercise. Also check whether the torso is flexing forward too much, as this may enhance stress on the low back. The lifter should look straight ahead, not toward the ceiling or elsewhere. Knees should not lock out at the top of the movement.

Comments & Suggestions: It is better to look straight ahead rather than looking up to the ceiling, as a forward gaze will help the lifter maintain balance. It is often recommended to keep the back "straight." Technically, this is incorrect because there is a natural curve in the human spinal cord. Instead, keep the back in a neutral position. Remember that inflexibility can limit ROM. Beginners usually squat incorrectly, pushing the knees past the toes. The often-recited advice of "pushing with the heels," which emphasizes the glutes more, may cause novices to lose balance and fall backward. Alternatively, try distributing the weight evenly over the feet at first. It is usually recommended not to squat below 90° because once the knees bend past this point, the stress on the joint increases dramatically. In theory, this may enhance or promote knee problems and pain. Dumbbell placement alters the feel of this exercise (e.g., dumbbells on shoulders vs. held at sides) and makes for good variations in this movement. This exercise can also be performed using a stability ball placed against a wall.

SQUAT WITH BARBELL

Primary Muscles Used: Quadriceps (vastus lateralis, vastus medialis, vastus intermedius, rectus femoris), hamstrings (semimembranosus, semitendinosus, biceps femoris), gluteal muscles.

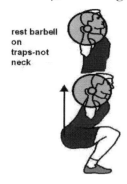

rest barbell on traps-not neck

> **Quick Tip:** Don't let knees go past toes. Look straight ahead—not upward at the ceiling.

Exercise Technique: Load an equally weighted barbell onto a power rack that has been adjusted to be at shoulder height or a little lower. This will allow the lifter to pick up and re-rack the weight more easily. Stand under the bar with feet about shoulder- or hip-width apart and pointed straight ahead. The bar should rest on the upper back and posterior deltoids near the trapezius and should be grasped a little wider than shoulder-width with a closed, pronated grip. In this position, the elbows are pointed outward from and behind the body to help keep the weight on the upper back. The weight should be evenly distributed over this area. Pull the shoulder blades together. The head looks straight ahead. Then, lift the weight upward by extending at the hips and knees. The barbell should rest freely on the upper body. Take a step or two backward in preparation for the eccentric phase of the lift. Feet are still about shoulder- to hip-width apart and toes pointed straight ahead.

Eccentric phase: Flex at the hips and knees and slowly lower the body, remembering not to lean too far forward. Stop the decent when the knees are flexed about 60–90° At this height, the thighs will be about parallel with the floor. Hold for 1 second.

Concentric phase: Extend at the hips and knees (as if getting up from a chair) to a standing position, being conscious not to lock out the knees at the top of the movement. Repeat for the desired number of repetitions.

Spotting: Ensure that the knees do not go past the toes and that the lifter does not descend lower than 90° or below the level at which he or she feels comfortable. If the heels come off of the floor, the lifter has gone too low for his or her level of flexibility. The knees should remain the same distance apart throughout the lift and should not bow inward or outward. Technically, at least two people should spot the squat—one on each end of the bar. This way, each spotter can cup his or her hands together and grasp the end of the barbell to easily help with lift-offs or whenever the lifter needs assistance.

Comments & Suggestions: The technique described here is different than for powerlifting and other competitive weightlifting events, where squatting lower than 90° may be necessary. Lower body flexibility impacts the ability to perform the squat and inflexibility can contribute to the compression forces felt on the spine. Placing blocks or weight plates under the heels can increase the stress on the knees.

Common Squat Mistakes

Mistake	Reason
Sacrificing form for weight lifted	Greatly enhances overall injury risk
Squatting below 90°	In theory, may increase risk of injury to knee joints
Resting barbell on cervical spine	Weight might fracture cervical spinal bones
Bouncing at bottom of exercise	Increases stress on knee joints and low back
Performing lifts too quickly	Increases overall injury risk
Knees traveling past toes	In theory, increases risk of injury to knee joints
Lifting too much weight	May activate GTO and muscle spindles, resulting in muscles relaxing when they are not supposed to. May increase risk of injury due to poor technique and overloading muscles before they are ready.
Looking upward to the ceiling	May cause neck strain or a loss of balance
Leaning too far forward	May cause loss of balance or neck injury
Toes turning inward	May lead to knee joint injury
Locking out knees	May lead to knee joint injury
Knees bowing inward	May lead to knee joint injury
Uneven gripping of barbell	May lead to loss of balance
Uneven placement of barbell	May lead to loss of balance
Heels coming off the ground	May lead to loss of balance
Bar placed too low on back	May increase stress on shoulders and increase chance of barbell rolling off back
Descending too fast	Lifter misses the advantages of eccentric muscle actions
Hands not pushing up on barbell	Increases risk that bar will slide off back

LUNGE (WITH DUMBBELLS)

Primary Muscles Used: Quadriceps (vastus lateralis, vastus medialis, vastus intermedius, rectus femoris), hamstrings (semimembranosus, semitendinosus, biceps femoris), gluteal muscles, calves (gastrocnemius, soleus).

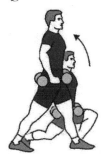

Quick Tip: Don't let knee travel in front of toes. Perform without dumbbells first.

Exercise Technique: Stand upright with weight evenly positioned over the feet. Feet should be about hip-width apart and pointed straight ahead. Hold equally weighted dumbbells at the sides with a neutral grip.

Eccentric phase: While keeping dumbbells close to the body, step forward so that there is no more than a 90° bend at the knee (the thigh will be parallel to the floor). The lifter's competency, balance, leg strength, and flexibility will dictate how far he or she can step forward with this exercise. The knee should not move from side to side but must stay in the same plane.

Concentric phase: Press the extended foot into the floor to lift the body back to the starting position. Repeat for the desired number of repetitions.

Spotting: Ensure that the forward knee does not travel beyond the toes and the shoulders do not travel past the hips. The lifter looks straight ahead. The trainer may be positioned to the side so that the lifter can hold onto the trainer's arm for added stability when learning this movement.

Comments & Suggestions: Practice with only bodyweight before incorporating resistances such as dumbbells. Be careful not to step too far forward at first, as this can reduce balance. This exercise can also be performed with a barbell or dumbbells placed at various positions to alter the difficulty of the exercise. If a barbell is used, make sure that it does not rest on the cervical spine. A variation of this exercise calls for the lifter to step backward (sometimes called a **reverse lunge**).

MACHINE SEATED LEG EXTENSION

Primary Muscles Used: Quadriceps (vastus lateralis, vastus medialis, vastus intermedius, rectus femoris).

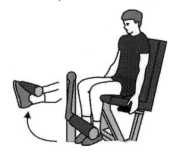

> **Quick Tip:** Align knee with rotational axis of machine.

Exercise Technique: Adjust the machine so that the knees are aligned with the axis of rotation and that the leg pads are positioned at the ankles. This usually requires adjusting the seat.

Concentric phase: Slowly raise legs as high as comfortable or until they reach the soft lockout position. Do not fully lock out the knees.

Eccentric phase: Slowly lower the legs to the starting position, halting just before the weight plates touch the weight stack. Repeat for the desired number of repetitions.

Spotting: Normally, the machine is adjusted so that the lifter starts with a 90° bend at the knees and aligns the knees with the rotational point of the machine. Ensure that the legs do not lock out at the top of the ROM. If the buttocks lift off of the seat during the eccentric phase, the weight is too heavy. The legs should move slowly during both concentric and eccentric phases with no quick or jerky movements. Likewise, the back should not arch during this movement.

Comments & Suggestions: While this exercise is usually performed with the toes pointed straight ahead, some research suggests that turning the toes inward recruits more of the outer quadriceps (vastus lateralis and vastus medialis) muscles, while pointing the toes outward places more stress on the inner quad and rectus femoris.[130] While toe positioning may isolate some muscle groups more than others, for most clients, pointing toes in different directions is not needed. Many perform this exercise with a 90° bend at the knee, although almost any ROM is possible, especially with machines that have adjustable ROM limiters. The lifter's goals, strength, and advice from a physical therapist (if applicable) will dictate the ROM of this exercise. Trainers should remember that greater stresses are placed on the knee joint when the leg is extended to full lockout. Thus, the higher one lifts, in theory, the greater the risk of knee injury. As such, a soft lockout is usually preferred. Because this is a single joint exercise, it is often wise to perform it after lower body multi-joint exercises like leg presses and squats. For added difficulty, perform this exercise using only one leg at a time.

Chondromalacia Patella

Chondromalacia patella, also known as "runner's knee," is a condition in which the kneecap is not properly aligned on the thighbone. The condition can occur following an injury, due to overuse, or without any specific injury at all. Weakness in the thighs or having flat feet may also contribute to the problem.[138] Common signs include pain behind the knee cap or behind the knee or pain felt while walking up or down stairs or after being seated for long periods of time.[133, 138] People may also feel sensations of grinding under the knee when they extend their leg.

Treatment often includes rest and icing the area as well as stretching the quadriceps, hamstrings, and calves. Warming up prior to activity can also help with pain. In addition, strengthening of the quadriceps may be required. If using a leg extension machine, adjust the machine so that that the leg only lifts up 6–8 inches before full leg extension occurs.[138] Alternatively, sit on the floor with the leg to be strengthened extended forward, then lift the straightened leg about 6–8 inches. Lower and repeat.

MACHINE SEATED HAMSTRING CURL

Primary Muscles Worked: Hamstrings (semimembranosus, semitendinosus, biceps femoris).

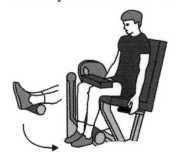

Quick Tip: Align knee with rotational axis of machine.

Exercise Technique: Sit in the machine with the legs over the leg pad. There should be a slight (10° to 20°) bend in the knees. If possible, adjust the lower leg pad so that it is positioned at the ankles, just above heels (at the Achilles tendon). The heels should be relaxed during the movement. Check to see that the middle and rear aspect of the knees are lined up with the axis of rotation of the machine. If not, adjust the seat. Note that the knees should remain lined up with the rotational point throughout the ROM. This may require testing with a light resistance first. The thigh support pad should also be in contact with the thighs (not the knees).

Concentric phase: Sitting upright in the machine with the buttocks pressed into the back pad, contract the abs. Then, in a controlled manner, slowly pull the legs downward, halting the movement at about 90° of knee flexion. At 90°, the lower legs will be perpendicular to the thighs. Hold the contraction for 1 second.

Eccentric phase: Slowly allow the legs to return to their starting position. Stop just before the weight plates of the machine touch. Repeat for the desired number of repetitions.

Spotting: Make sure that the middle part of the knee is aligned with the machine's axis of rotation during the ROM. This is most easily seen when kneeling off to the side of the machine. The rotation axis can sometimes be identified by a small colored dot or plastic cup that covers or highlights the axis. Make sure that the toes do not rotate outward or inward, as this may increase stress on the knee.

Comments & Suggestions: Failure of the lifter to sit upright in the machine may be a sign of hamstring inflexibility. Some machines of this type start the ROM with the feet higher than the knees, which puts the knee in a hyper-flexed position. In theory, this may increase the risk of knee injury. The seated leg curl machine is usually preferable to the prone version, particularly for people with heart disease and high blood pressure. Many machines have numbers on the seat to help clients remember their settings. This can help trainers who design programs for people whom they see infrequently. This exercise can also be performed with a stability ball for added difficulty.

MACHINE PRONE HAMSTRING CURL

Primary Muscles Worked: Hamstrings (semimembranosus, semitendinosus, biceps femoris).

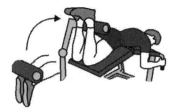

Quick Tip: Align knee with rotational axis of machine. People with heart disease may get dizzy if they rise too quickly from this machine.

Exercise Technique: Adjust the weight stack to the desired resistance. Adjust the ankle pad (if possible) so that it rests above the heels. Lay face down (prone) on the machine with the legs under the ankle pad. In this position, the knees should have a slight (10–20°) bend in them. If the machine has handgrips, grasp them lightly. The knees should be slightly off of the pad. The knees should also be lined up with the rotational axis of the machine. A small, colored circular dot or plastic cup may highlight this area. The feet should be relaxed.

Concentric phase: Slowly the lift legs until a 90° bend at the knee is reached (at 90°, the ankles will point straight up).

Eccentric phase: Slowly lower to the starting position, halting just before the weight stack touches the other weight plates. Do not lock out the knees at the end of the eccentric phase. Repeat for the desired number of repetitions.

Spotting: Make sure that the hips do not come off of the machine, as this may stress the low back. Angled benches make this less likely, but it may still happen. The knees should be off of the edge of the thigh pad, not pressed into the pad. There should be a slight bend at the knees when the legs are extended. The middle part of the knees should be aligned with the rotational axis of the machine. Do not let the lifter's head arch up during this exercise.

Comments & Suggestions: Because more tension is placed on the hamstrings in the prone position, this exercise may work the hamstrings a bit more than the seated version. By the same token, this movement may be more difficult for those with tight hamstrings. It is not necessary for the ankle pad to touch the buttocks at the end of the concentric phase. People with heart disease and/or blood pressure issues may become dizzy if they rise too quickly, as this movement may cause a temporary drop in blood pressure (called orthostatic hypotension). This may result in falls. For these individuals and for people with back problems, the seated version may be a safer alternative. The seated version is probably better for clients you only see occasionally as well.

HAMSTRING CURL WITH STABILITY BALL

Primary Muscles Used: Hamstrings (semimembranosus, semitendinosus, biceps femoris).

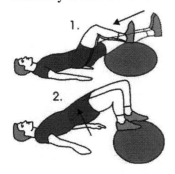

> **Quick Tip:** Keep the buttocks elevated during the exercise. Bringing the arms closer to the sides increases the difficulty.

Exercise Technique: Obtain a stability ball and lie supine on the floor. Extend the legs and place the tops of the heels or ankles on the ball. Extend the arms out to the sides to about 45° to aid with stability. Extend the hips by pressing the heels and ankles into the ball and lifting the buttocks off of the floor with the legs extended. Maintain a slight bend in the knees.

Concentric phase: Slowly draw the ball inward toward the buttocks by bending the knees. Hold for 1 second.

Eccentric phase: Move the ball away by extending the legs. Stop when there is a slight bend at the knees. Repeat for the desired number of repetitions.

Spotting: The hips and buttocks should remain elevated and the body should not wobble while performing the exercise. The head should remain on the floor.

Comments & Suggestions: To learn this movement, it may be necessary to first strengthen the core by performing with calves on ball and by only raising the buttocks into air. Because this exercise uses the stability ball, more than the hamstrings are being utilized. Other muscles involved include the calves as well as the abs and back muscles. While keeping the hips elevated is important, it is not necessary to thrust the hips upward as shown in this picture. That is an advanced form of the exercise and can be a future goal.

SEATED OUTER THIGH MACHINE

Primary Muscles Used: Gluteus medius, gluteus minimus, tensor fasciae latae.

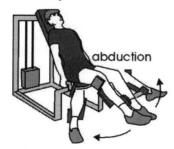

> **Quick Tip:** The outer part of the knee should be lined up with the kneepads.

Exercise Technique: The exercise is started with the legs inside the kneepads and the legs close to each other. The kneepads should be placed against the outer part of the knees. In some versions, the knees are bent 90°. Some versions also have a place to rest the feet during the exercise.

Concentric phase: Slowly press against the leg pads and open the legs to a comfortable position. Hold for 1 second.

Eccentric phase: Slowly lower to the starting position, stopping just before the weight stack touches. Repeat.

Spotting: The low back should not arch during the exercise.

Comments & Suggestions: The technical name for this exercise is **hip abduction** because the hips are abducting (moving away) from the body. Physical and occupational therapists often say "AB-duction" so that it is not confused with "ADD-duction" ("adding" or moving the body part toward the body." It is a myth that this exercise reduces body fat from the sides of the hips.

SEATED INNER THIGH MACHINE

Primary Muscles Used: Gracillis, adductor longus, adductor magnus, adductor brevis, pectineus.

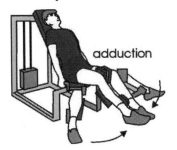

> **Quick Tip:** The inner part of the knees should be lined up with the kneepads.

Exercise Technique: If necessary, first adjust the machine so that the kneepads are close together. Sit in the machine with the inner knees aligned with the kneepads. Rest the feet on the foot supports (if applicable). Then, open the legs to a comfortable position, which for many people is when they feel a slight pull in their inner thighs. If the low back arches, the legs are open too widely.

Concentric phase: Slowly close the legs by pressing the knees against the kneepads until the kneepads touch each other. Hold for second.

Eccentric phase: Slowly release the tension, opening the legs to the starting position. Repeat. At the end of the set, readjust the kneepads so that they are close together to make it easier to exit the machine.

Spotting: The low back should not arch during the exercise. Both the concentric and eccentric phases should be performed in a slow, controlled manner. Letting the legs open quickly while under tension may result in injury.

Comments & Suggestions: Adduction (or "AD-duction") refers to moving a body part closer to the midline of the body. While this exercise can strengthen the inner thigh muscles, it is a myth that it burns fat from the inner thighs. For most people, it is not necessary to open the legs more than about 45° before starting the movement. This exercise can also be performed by squeezing a stability ball between the legs.

HIP EXTENSION WITH MULTI-HIP MACHINE

Primary Muscles Used: Hamstrings (semimembranosus, semitendinosus, biceps femoris), gluteus maximus.

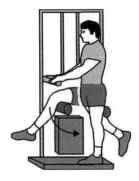

> **Quick Tip:** The upper body should not lean forward or backward during the exercise.

Exercise Technique: Adjust the machine so that the hip is lined up with the rotational point of the machine. Adjust the kneepad so that it is elevated and behind the knee of the leg that is exercised, as shown in the picture. The other leg should be slightly bent at the knee. The hands should lightly grasp the stabilizing arm of the machine for support.

Concentric phase: Slowly bring the leg backward, halting when it is past the stationary leg.

Eccentric phase: Slowly release the tension until the leg is at its starting position. Repeat for the desired number of repetitions.

Spotting: The upper body should not lean forward or backward during the exercise. The hip should be aligned with the rotational axis of the machine. The head should look forward and not turn to the sides.

Comments & Suggestions: How far one presses backward during the concentric phase depends on his or her ability to stay upright in a neutral position. In theory, this exercise may exacerbate low back problems in some individuals.

STIFF LEG DEAD LIFT

Primary Muscled Used: Hamstrings (semimembranosus, semitendinosus, biceps femoris), gluteal muscles, erector spinae.

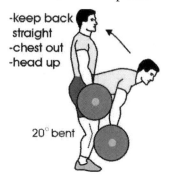

-keep back straight
-chest out
-head up

20° bent

Quick Tip: Keep the weight close to the body and do not lock out the knees.

Exercise Technique: Obtain an equally weighted Olympic bar or barbell and stand over it with the feet about shoulder to hip-width apart. The feet should be either pointed straight ahead or slightly angled outward. Squat down and grasp the bar with a closed, pronated grip about shoulder-width apart. In this position, the back should be firm and arched slightly and the chest should be oriented forward and upward. The head should be elevated slightly.

Concentric phase: Pull the shoulder blades together and lift the barbell upward, keeping it close to the body. At the top of the ROM, the knees should be slightly flexed (about 20°).

Eccentric phase: Slowly lower the barbell by bending at the hips while maintaining a slight bend in the knees. The back stays neutral and rigid and the shoulders remain pinched together to prevent them from being rounded forward. The descent stops if the heels come off of the floor or when the lifter feels a contraction in the hamstrings. Repeat.

Spotting: It is important that the weight remain very close to the body at all times. Failure to do so increases injury risk. Ensure that the shoulders do not round forward. In general, the shoulders should not be lower than the hips during the decent phase. Flexing so far that the torso is parallel with the ground greatly increases low back injury risk. Sometimes, lifters flex at the wrists, but this is improper technique. No bouncing or exploding upward during the movement should occur, as this increases injury risk. The spine should not hyperextend during the ascent phase.

Comments & Suggestions: Lifers sometimes call stiff leg deadlifts "stiffies," but this does not mean that the knees are stiff in a lockout stance. Rather, a slight bend is maintained at the knee during this movement. This exercise can also be performed with dumbbells or, in the case of beginners, with no weight at all.

This is a complicated movement. Bending at the waist, especially when holding an external resistance, places the low back under a lot of stress and greatly enhances the injury risk to the spinal disks of the low back.[132] If performed incorrectly, this movement can cause injury.[132] Lifters should have a strong foundation in strength training and have very good flexibility in the hamstrings and back before attempting. This exercise is not for beginners. Some lifters perform this movement while standing on an exercise bench to obtain a greater ROM. This further increases injury risk and should not be performed. This movement should not be performed by those with current or former injuries to the low back. Likewise, the movement might exacerbate injuries to the knees, neck, or shoulders.

DEADLIFT WITH BARBELL

Primary Muscles Worked: Gluteus maximus, hamstrings (semimembranosus, semitendinosus, biceps femoris), erector spinae, quadriceps (vastus lateralis, vastus intermedius, vastus medialis, rectus femoris), rhomboids, trapezius, deltoids.

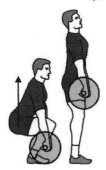

> **Quick Tip:** Keep the weight close to the body at all times.

Exercise Technique: Load an Olympic bar (or barbell) with equal weight on each side. The lifter's feet should be between shoulder- and hip-width apart and pointed straight ahead or slightly outward. The lifter squats and grasps the bar with an alternated grip that is slightly wider than shoulder-width apart. The back is stiff and rigid. The shoulder blades should be retracted and the chest oriented upward. In this position, the shoulders will be slightly over the barbell.

Concentric phase: Slowly lift the barbell upward by extending the hips and knees while keeping the weight evenly distributed over the feet. The chest is still oriented upward. Continue the lift until standing straight up with a soft lockout at the knees. Do not hyperextend the back. The barbell should be close to the body throughout the movement.

Eccentric phase: Flex at the hips and knees, lowering the barbell to the floor while simultaneously keeping it close to the body. Touch the floor lightly with the barbell while keeping tension in the muscles in preparation for the next concentric action. Repeat.

Spotting: Ensure that the knees do not travel past the toes and that the shoulders do not round forward. The head should look straight ahead or slightly upward.

Comments & Suggestions: The deadlift is a complicated movement. As such, lifters should first develop a good strength base before progressing to this exercise. The weight should be evenly balanced over the feet. While an alternated grip is used in this example, a pronated grip can also be used.

Basic Knee Safety Guidelines

Warm up first	Do not lift too much weight
Do not lock out the knees. Do not let the knees travel past toes.	Do not bounce at the bottom of the movement (e.g., during squats)
Align knees with rotation axis of machine (e.g., in the leg extension machine)	Do not turn the toes inward
Do not place blocks or weight plates under the heels	Do not let the knees make contact with ground (e.g., during lunges)

Basic Low Back Safety Guidelines

Warm up first	Retract shoulder blades with heavy lifts. Do not round shoulders. Keep weight close to body.
Bend and lift with knees and hips, not with the back	Maintain strong abdominals
Maintain flexibility in hamstrings	Maintain flexibility in quadriceps
Maintain strength in low back muscles	Do not arch the back

SEATED CALF RAISE

Primary Muscles Used: Soleus (gastrocnemius, to a lesser extent).

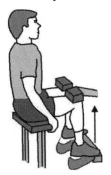

> **Quick Tip:** Determine flexibility in the calves before adding weight to the machine.

Exercise Technique: Sit straight up in the machine with knees bent to 90° and the thigh pad just behind the knees, resting on the thighs. In this position, the ankles should be perpendicular to the floor. The balls of the feet should be on the raised foot platform. The exercise is started when the calves are supporting the weight, after the load has been removed from its resting location.

Concentric phase: Elevate the calves as high as is comfortable.

Eccentric phase: Slowly lower the weight until the heels are at least level with the toes or a little below this point. Repeat for the desired number of repetitions.

Spotting: Check that the toes do not slide off of the elevated foot platform and that the thigh pad is not compressing the knees. Handgrips are usually present on these machines, and the hands should rest comfortably yet not grasp them tightly or pull up on them. The knees and toes should stay pointed straight ahead throughout the ROM.

Comments & Suggestions: Both the soleus and gastrocnemius play roles in ankle stability and balance. These muscles may also be weak after ACL surgery.[134] The big difference between this exercise and the standing calf raise is that this movement works more of the soleus muscle while the standing calf raise targets more of the gastrocnemius. Because of variations in calf flexibility, this exercise is safest if the trainer first assesses how far the heels can lower without any resistance. Sometimes people train calves using a leg press machine—this particular exercise works mostly the gastrocnemius because the legs are straight. If no machine is available, the seated calf raise can also be performed in a chair with dumbbells resting on the thighs.

STANDING CALF RAISE WITH DUMBBELL

Primary Muscles Used: Gastrocnemius.

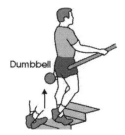

Dumbbell

Quick Tip: Determine how low the heel can go before adding additional weight.

Exercise Technique: Obtain a dumbbell and stand on a step with the balls of the feet at the edge. The dumbbell should be held on the same side as the ankle to be worked. The other hand can be used for support. The foot is pointed straight ahead and there is a slight bend at the knee.

Eccentric phase: Slowly lower the heel until tension is felt.

Concentric phase: Rise up to the starting position or higher, depending on ankle strength. Repeat.

Spotting: The knee should not be locked out. Ensure that the toes do not slide off of the step during the movement. The upper body should stay neutral and neither hyperextend backward nor flex forward. The head should remain neutral and not turn to the sides.

Comments & Suggestions: Both the gastrocnemius and soleus are involved in plantar flexion (raising the heel upward). Together, both muscles form a muscle group that is sometimes called the **triceps surae**. One difference between the two muscles is that the gastrocnemius is made up mostly of type II muscle fibers, while the soleus is composed mainly of type I.[135] In this exercise, the gastrocnemius is the main muscle targeted. During the seated version, on the other hand, the soleus works more. It is safest to first determine flexibility in the calf before adding weight. The normal progression for this movement is to first perform with two feet with no added weight.

SPIDER CURLS WITH BARBELL

Primary Muscles Used: Biceps.

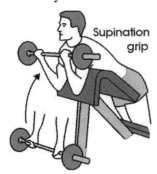

Supination grip

Quick Tip: Pull shoulder blades together and keep the elbows pointed straight ahead.

Exercise Technique: Obtain a barbell and lean against the opposite side of a preacher curl bench. Performed this way, the back of the arms will rest against the pad against which the chest normally presses. The hands should be about shoulder-width apart and the feet are placed about hip- to shoulder-width apart, while the wrists remain neutral and do not bend. Pull the shoulder blades together to aid with shoulder stabilization.

Eccentric phase: With a closed, supinated grip, slowly lower the barbell until it is almost straight down, (i.e., to a soft lockout position).

Concentric phase: Lift the barbell until it is between 90–120°.

Spotting: The head should stay neutral and not become hyperextended. The shoulders should stay neutral and not round forward. The elbows should not flair outward or inward. Hand the barbell to the lifter after he or she assumes the appropriate position. Remove the barbell when the lifter has finished the set.

Comments & Suggestions: This is a variation of a preacher curl. The advantage of this variation is that it allows the muscle to be worked against gravity over a greater ROM. It can also be performed laying face down on an incline bench. Because of the angle, the lifter will likely need to use less weight than on other biceps exercises. This exercise might exacerbate low back pain. It can also be performed with dumbbells or an EZ curl bar. If working out at home, the back of a kitchen chair can also be used for support.

STANDING BICEPS CURL WITH BARBELL

Primary Muscles Worked: Biceps group, brachioradialis.

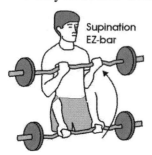

Supination
EZ-bar

> **Quick Tip:** Raise the barbell to only 90°. Don't let the elbows drift forward during the exercise.

Exercise Technique: Grasp an equally weighted barbell with a closed, supinated grip. The grip should be shoulder-width apart or a little wider. The knees are slightly bent and the feet are about shoulder- to hip-width apart.

Concentric phase: With the elbows aligned under the shoulders, slowly raise the barbell until it is at about 90° or, if preferred, almost to the height of the shoulders.

Eccentric phase: Slowly lower the barbell to the starting position, halting just before the elbows fully lock out. Repeat.

Spotting: This exercise is usually spotted from behind so that the trainer can ensure that the elbows do not move from the sides of the body, although spotting from the front is okay as well. The lifter's body should not rock back and forth during the exercise. The shoulders should not shrug upward. Ensure that there is a slight bend in the knees and that the abs are slightly contracted. Make sure that the weight is lowered slowly to take full advantage of the eccentric action.

Comments & Suggestions: While an EZ curl bar is shown here, a straight barbell can also be used, as can dumbbells. People often ask which is better for developing the biceps—the straight bar or an EZ curl bar. While few head-to-head comparisons appear in peer-reviewed journals, the straight bar barbell probably outperforms the EZ curl bar in this author's opinion. Anatomically, this has to do with the two functions of the biceps—elbow flexion and supination. By holding the straight bar while curling the barbell, one also has his or her hands supinated. By combining both actions of the biceps, one probably puts a greater stress on that muscle. With the EZ curl bar, on the other hand, the hands are not as supinated. This allows for the other muscles of the arm (such as the brachioradialis and radials) to help. The EZ curl bar, however, does have its place, and performing either of these variations alone is probably not as effective as incorporating both.

Because a barbell is a free weight, it opposes gravity, which always acts downward. Thus, the biceps are maximally contracted (and maximally working against gravity) when the arm is curled to only 90°. Lifting the weight more than this is not wrong, but for those who normally lift through a greater ROM, performing only to 90° will add nice variety and a challenging element to this exercise.

Because the biceps are used in most pulling exercises, a good case can be made that this muscle group is overemphasized in most fitness programs.

MACHINE BICEPS CURL

Primary Muscles Worked: Biceps group, brachioradialis.

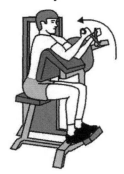

> **Quick Tip:** Align elbows with rotation point of machine.

Exercise Technique: Adjust the seat such that the backs of the arms are supported on the arm pads of the machine. The middle portion of the elbows should also be aligned with the rotation point of the machine. Grasp the handles with a closed, supinated grip. The elbows should have a slight bend and not be locked out. The chest and upper torso should rest against the chest pad of the machine.

Concentric phase: Contract the biceps and slowly lift until the handles are close to the shoulders or until the position feels comfortable. The wrists should not be bent.

Eccentric phase: Lower the weight in a controlled manner until there is a slight bend in elbows. Repeat.

Spotting: The elbows should be aligned with the rotational point of the machine throughout the ROM. The lifter should not rock back and forth or hunch the shoulders as the weight is lifted.

Comments & Suggestions: Some versions of this machine allow the hands to rotate from a pronated (palms facing down) position to a full supination (palms up) position during the ROM. Supination brings the biceps into action more than pronation. Biceps curls may exacerbate elbow injuries such as tendonitis. Use caution in those with osteoporosis, as some versions of this machine may cause excessive forward trunk flexion that may increase the risk of spinal fractures. Because this machine does not rely on gravity for resistance, a greater resisted ROM is possible than with free weights. On the downside, this is an isolation exercise that uses fewer muscles than a standing barbell or dumbbell curl. With some versions of this machine, it is possible to curl the weight up so far that it may impact the head, so exercise caution.

STANDING CABLE BICEPS CURL

Primary Muscles Used: Biceps, brachioradialis.

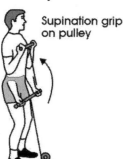

Supination grip on pulley

Quick Tip: Keep elbows at sides at all times. For a variation, perform while supine on the floor.

Exercise Technique: Stand facing a selectorized cable machine. Grasp handles using a supine, closed grip. The elbows remain at the sides and do not move throughout the ROM. The knees are about hip- to shoulder-width apart and have a slight bend. Abs are slightly contracted and the shoulder blades are retracted.

Concentric phase: Slowly lift weight, stopping at about 90° or a little higher.

Eccentric phase: Slowly lower the weight in a controlled manner until there is a slight bend in the elbows. Repeat.

Spotting: Ensure that the upper body does not rock back and forth during the exercise and that the elbows do not move forward in front of the body. The knees should remain in a soft lockout position throughout the ROM.

Comments & Suggestions: Because of diversity in design, the same resistance can feel very different among machines. People sometimes try to fight the resistance by bringing the elbows forward, in front of the body, which takes the stress off of the biceps and may contribute to the development of tennis elbow. Arching of the back is also possible and this, too, should be avoided. This exercise places less stress on the low back if performed supine.

HAMMER CURL WITH DUMBBELLS

Primary Muscles Worked: Brachialis, brachioradialis.

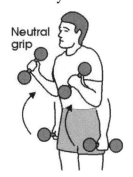

Neutral grip

> **Quick Tip:** For added difficulty, lift dumbbells only to 90°.

Exercise Technique: This exercise can be performed while standing or sitting. Grasp two equally weighted dumbbells. The dumbbells should be held with a neutral grip throughout the exercise.

Concentric phase. Slowly raise the dumbbells to about 90° while keeping the elbows at the sides. The forearms will be parallel to the floor.

Eccentric phase. Slowly lower to a point just before the elbows lock out fully. Repeat for the desired number of repetitions. If performed standing, the feet should be about hip- to shoulder-width apart and there should be a slight bend in the knees.

Spotting: This exercise is usually spotted from behind so that the trainer can ensure that the elbows do not move from the sides of the body, although spotting from the front is also acceptable. The lifter's body should not rock back and forth during the exercise and the shoulders should not shrug upward. Make certain that there is a slight bend in the knees and that the abs are contracted. The weight should be lowered slowly to take advantage of the eccentric phase.

Comments & Suggestions: The neutral grip places less emphasis on the biceps group, so this exercise is sometimes overlooked. However, the muscles targeted in this movement can also help with overall biceps development. Remember, there is more to the upper arm than the biceps.

TRICEPS PUSHDOWN

Primary Muscles Used: Triceps.

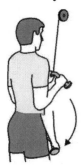

> **Quick Tip:** Keep the elbows held to the sides of the body at all times.

Exercise Technique: Stand facing the machine and grasp the bar with a closed, pronated grip. The grip used can vary from very close to wide. The feet should be hip- to shoulder-width apart. The knees should be slightly flexed and there should be a slight forward lean at the hips, such that the bodyweight is aligned over the ankles. Stand close enough so that the cable hangs straight down when the exercise is performed. Pull the bar down until the arms are bent at about 90° and the elbows are tucked into the sides of the body. At this point, the upper arms are pointed straight down and the forearms are parallel to floor.

Concentric phase: Slowly press downward until the arms are almost straight (i.e., to a soft lockout position). Hold for 1 second.

Eccentric phase: Slowly release the tension, raising the bar back up to the starting position. Repeat.

Spotting: A very common mistake is letting the elbows move forward and away from the sides of body. This takes the stress off of the triceps. To address this, place towels between the torso and elbows or touch the lifter's elbows with your fingers so that the elbows remain stationary at the sides of the body. Make sure that the hands are evenly spaced on the bar. Two other common mistakes are bending the wrists and turning the head. Rocking back and forth may occur with heavy resistances and should be discouraged.

Comments & Suggestions: Some people perform this exercise while standing straight up at attention. With heavier resistances, though, this practice can place undue stress on the low back. Bending at the hips and knees reduces this risk. Some cable machines allow this exercise to be performed with one's back pressed against the machine, which may be better for those with back issues. While a semi-pronated grip is depicted here, a straight bar or a rope can also be used. If a rope is used, the weight lifted may feel heaver than when a metal bar is used because the rope is lighter and there is less of a counterweight effect. Because this is a single joint exercise, lifting maximum loads (e.g., 1RM) is not recommended.

TRICEPS EXTENSION MACHINE

Primary Muscles Used: Triceps.

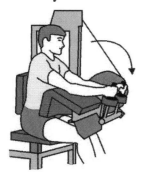

> **Quick Tip:** The upper arms should stay on the arm pad during the upward, eccentric phase of the exercise.

Exercise Technique: Adjust the seat of the machine so that the upper arms are at about shoulder height and the elbows are aligned with the rotational point of the machine. The upper arms should be pointing up toward the ceiling (i.e., the elbows should be bent about 90°). The chest should be against the chest pad of the machine (on some versions) and the back in a neutral position (neither hunched forward nor hyperextended backward).

Concentric phase: Grasp the handles with a neutral grip (palms facing each other) and press forward and downward, halting just before the elbows are completely locked out. Hold for 1 second.

Eccentric phase: Slowly release the tension, returning to the starting position. Repeat.

Spotting: Make sure that the elbows are aligned with the machine's axis of rotation. Neither the elbows nor the upper arms should come off of the arm pad during the eccentric phase.

Comments & Suggestions: Some versions allow for each arm to be used independently. This exercise can also be performed lying supine with dumbbells or with a standing triceps pushdown.

TRICEPS KICKBACK WITH DUMBBELL

Primary Muscles Used: Triceps.

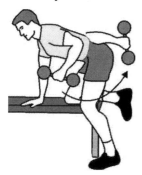

> **Quick Tip**: Keep the upper arm parallel to the floor.

Exercise Technique: Hold a dumbbell with one hand and place the knee of the opposite side of the body on a stable exercise bench. The dumbbell should be held with a neutral grip during the exercise. Bend forward at the hips and place the other hand on the bench for support. The other leg remains on the floor with the knee slightly bent. Abs stay tight throughout the entire movement. Generally, the upper torso should be angled slightly upward to about 30–45° when in this position. Bend the elbow of the hand holding the dumbbell to 90° and hold the upper arm close to the side of the body, making it about parallel to the floor.

Concentric phase: Press the dumbbell upward and backward by extending the elbow, while keeping the upper arm stationary at the side of the body. Do not completely lock out the elbow at the top of the movement. Hold for 1 second.

Eccentric phase: Slowly lower to the starting position, stopping when the forearm is pointing straight down. Repeat.

Spotting: The head should remain neutral. If the wrists bend downward, the weight is too heavy.

Comments & Suggestions: It is not necessary to bring the dumbbell close to the anterior shoulder during the eccentric phase. This engages the brachialis and biceps, which are not the targeted muscles of this exercise. Because of the angle involved, less weight will be used in comparison with other triceps exercises. Because triceps are involved in pressing movements, they tend to be overemphasized in most exercise programs.

SUPINE TRICEPS EXTENSION WITH DUMBBELLS

Primary Muscles Used: Triceps.

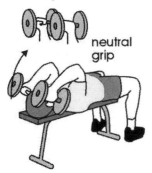

neutral
grip

> **Quick Tip:** Upper arms should point upward to ceiling during this movement.

Exercise Technique: Obtain two equally weighted dumbbells and recline supine on a stable exercise bench as shown. The feet should be about hip- to shoulder-width apart. The exercise begins with the arms extended (with a slight bend in the elbows) and dumbbells held over the chest.

Eccentric phase: Slowly lower dumbbells toward the forehead or just past it while keeping the upper arms pointed upward toward the ceiling. Stop when there is about a 90° bend at the elbows.

Concentric phase: Slowly raise dumbbells to starting position, halting just before the elbows lock out. Repeat.

Spotting: The upper arms should be perpendicular to the floor throughout the movement. The low back should not arch upward and the feet should remain on the floor. If the back arches, rest the feet on a stable box or exercise step. Placement of the feet on the exercise bench is also possible, but this increases the balance requirement of the exercise. Make sure that the lifter does not lose his or her grip on the dumbbells. At no time should the dumbbells make contact with the head.

Comments & Suggestions: This exercise is also called the "skull crusher" because of the possibility of what can happen if the exercise is not performed correctly. Some lifers use a variety of grips when training the triceps (including supinated, neutral, and pronated grips). While it does not appear that one grip activates the triceps more than another, altering the grip adds variety and, in theory, may reduce the prevalence of overuse injuries.

Triceps Tendonitis

Triceps tendonitis results from an inflammation of the triceps tendon, which is located behind the elbow on the upper arm. It can result from overuse (doing too many chest and triceps exercises) or from overloading the muscles faster than they can adjust.[133] Symptoms can include pain, redness, or warmth over the back of the elbow. Treatment often includes ice, rest, stretching, and eventually strengthening of both the triceps and biceps, which work together to keep the elbow structurally sound.[133] If the condition persists for more than two weeks without improvement, a referral to a physician or physical therapist is warranted.

MODIFIED SUPERMAN

Primary Muscles Used: Gluteus maximus, hamstrings, rectus abdominis, internal and external obliques, deltoids, rhomboids, trapezius.

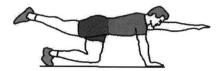

Quick Tip: For added difficulty, try performing on a stability ball.

Exercise Technique: The exercise begins when the person supports his or her body weight with both hands and knees on the floor. Prior to the exercise, the arms should be in line with the shoulders and the knees in line with the hips. The head and trunk should be neutral, about parallel to the floor. The abs should be slightly contracted.

Performing the exercise: Simultaneously raise the right arm and left leg slowly until they are at about trunk level. Hold for 1–2 seconds and lower to the starting position. Then, lift the left arm and right leg until they are level with the trunk. Lower to the starting position. Alternate the limbs like this for the desired number of repetitions.

Spotting: The head stays neutral, neither looking upward nor to the sides. The low back should not slouch downward.

Comments & Suggestions: The superman exercise occurs when the person is prone on the floor or bench and lifts the arms and legs upward at the same time. This modified version recruits more of the core musculature and is a good movement to enhance overall core stabilization. Those with weaker core muscles may have a smaller ROM—this is okay. Progress slowly as strength improves. For an added challenge, do not alternate limbs but rather perform all the repetitions on one side before moving to the other side. Another name for this exercise is the "quadruped."

BACK EXTENSION WITH STABILITY BALL

Primary Muscles Worked: Erector spinae.

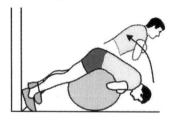

Quick Tip: For added difficulty, don't anchor the feet to the wall.

Exercise Technique: Obtain a stability ball and lie face down on the ball with the belly button positioned near or at the top of the ball. The legs are hip- to shoulder-width apart and extended. There should be a slight bend in the knees. The feet can be pressed against a wall or ankles held by the trainer for added stability. The hands can be held at the sides, crossed over the chest, or stretched forward, depending on the level of difficulty desired. Before the exercise begins, the lifter's trunk is flexed, which facilitates the upward concentric action.

Concentric phase: Retract the shoulder blades and slowly lift the upper body upward until it is approximately in line with the legs.

Eccentric phase: Slowly lower to starting position. Repeat for the desired number of repetitions.

Spotting: Ensure that the shoulder blades remain retracted throughout the movement. The head should stay neutral. If stabilizing the lifter, the trainer should hold the client's ankles.

Comments & Suggestions: It is not necessary to hyperextend the back on this exercise. Also, for many people, it is not necessary to use added resistance, as most people can be adequately challenged using body weight only. For most healthy people, several sets of 15–20 repetitions should be mastered before an external resistance is used. Back extensions may be inappropriate for people with back injuries. If this exercise hurts, try the modified superman described previously. For added difficulty, perform with the feet not anchored to a wall or supported by a trainer.

REVERSE BACK EXTENSION WITH STABILTY BALL

Primary Muscles Used: Erector spinae, gluteus maximus, hamstrings.

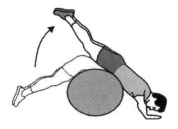

> **Quick Tip:** Begin with a small range of motion. Also try with knees bent.

Exercise Technique: Lie prone on a stability ball so that the head is lower than the hips. In this position, the ball will be at about hip level. At this point, the feet may either be slightly off of the floor or just touching it. The legs should be extended but slightly bent at the knees, about hip-width apart. The head remains neutral and hands stay on the floor facing forward, about shoulder-width apart. The abs are tight.

Concentric phase: Contract the glutes and slowly raise the legs upward until comfortable or until they are in line with body. This is usually about 45°. Hold for 1 second.

Eccentric phase: Slowly lower the legs to the starting point. Repeat for the desired number of repetitions.

Spotting: The motion should be slow and controlled with no momentum used to swing or bounce the legs upward. The legs should go no higher than the hips. Going further than this may cause the low back to hyperextend.

Comments & Suggestions: This exercise can also be performed with bent knees. It is important to do this exercise slowly, using little momentum. This exercise can also be performed on a bench if a stability ball is not available. Rise up slowly after completing because of possible temporary drops in blood pressure in some individuals.

CRUNCH ON STABILITY BALL

Primary Muscles Used: Rectus abdominis, internal and external obliques.

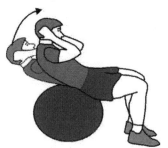

> **Quick Tip:** For added difficulty, try performing with one leg in the air.

Exercise Technique: Recline supine on a stability ball with the feet about shoulder-width apart and knees bent to about 90°. When the individual is supine, the ball should rest somewhere between the low- to middle-back range, depending on fitness level and difficulty desired.

Concentric phase: Contract the abs and slowly curl the torso upward, bringing the ribs closer to the hips.

Eccentric phase: Slowly lower to the starting point. Repeat for the desired number of repetitions.

Spotting: The upper torso should curl inward and become concave as it is lifted. Clasping the hands behind the neck may increase neck strain.

Comments & Suggestions: It is not necessary to curl all the way up to a seated upright position on the ball—just a slight movement is all that is needed to challenge the abs. If this exercise is performed slowly, the abs should be sufficiently challenged after 12–20 repetitions. There are many ways to increase the difficulty of this exercise. For example, extending the arms over and behind the head or performing with one leg in the air increases the difficulty, as does placing the ball closer to the lower back area. Some research suggests that greater abdominal recruitment occurs when the ball is placed closer to the low back region relative to performing crunches on the floor.[139] It is a myth that crunches selectively burn fat from the belly area.

REVERSE CRUNCH WITH STABILITY BALL

Primary Muscles Used: Rectus abdominis, internal and external obliques.

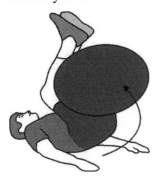

> **Quick Tip:** For added difficulty, this can also be performed with different sized stability balls or with a medicine ball.

Exercise Technique: Obtain a stability ball and recline supine with legs bent over the ball about shoulder-width apart. The back of the heels should press into the ball to aid in the lifting process. The arms should be at the sides with the hands facing down.

Concentric phase: Contract the abdominals and slowly lift the ball into the air until comfortable or until the buttocks is slightly off of the floor.

Eccentric phase: Slowly lower the ball until it is almost touching the ground. Repeat for the desired number of repetitions.

Spotting: The head should be neutral. The low back should not come off the floor. If the ball touches the floor, it reduces tension on the abdominals.

Comments & Suggestions: Become proficient at performing the movement without a stability ball first. For added difficulty, lift the shoulders off of the ground at the same time that the ball is lifted. It is very easy for the hip flexors to do all of the work on this exercise, especially when it is performed at a fast pace. Focus on working the abdominals.

OBLIQUE CRUNCH ON STABILITY BALL

Primary Muscles Used: Rectus abdominis, internal and external obliques, erector spinae.

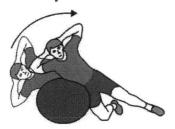

> **Quick Tip:** Placing the feet against a wall makes this exercise easier.

Exercise Technique: Recline sideways on the stability ball as shown, with the ball positioned at the midsection. The legs are extended with the inner leg behind the outer leg and flexed to aid with support. The outer leg should also be slightly bent.

Concentric phase: Slowly lift the body upward, bringing the ribs closer to the hips. Hold for 1 second.

Eccentric phase: Slowly lower the body to the starting position. Repeat for the desired number of repetitions.

Spotting: The body should be centered equally on the ball. The head should be neutral.

Comments & Suggestions: Some recommend that the inner leg be extended with the outer leg behind it. Experiment to find which leg position works best for you. This is a challenging movement because less of the body remains in contact with the ball. Bringing the legs closer increases the difficulty of this exercise. For more stability, perform with feet against a wall. This exercise does not selectively target fat loss from the sides of the abs, also known as the "love handles."

PRONE KNEE TUCK WITH STABILITY BALL

Primary Muscles Used: Abdominals (rectus abdominis, internal and external obliques), core musculature.

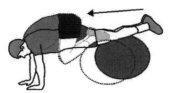

Quick Tip: The exercise is harder when the ball is closer to the toes and even more difficult if performed with only one leg.

Exercise Technique: Obtain a stability ball and lie prone on it. Walk outward with your arms and hands so that you are in a push-up position. At this point, the ball should be near the middle thighs.

Concentric phase: Slowly bend at the hips and knees, pulling the knees toward the chest, moving the ball closer to the body.

Eccentric phase: Slowly extend the legs so that the ball moves back to its starting point. Repeat for the desired number of repetitions.

Spotting: The low back should not drop downward toward the floor during this movement. The head should be neutral. The hands should be about shoulder-width apart and oriented forward.

Comments & Suggestions: This exercise requires much upper body strength and balance. First, practice learning how to roll out and back on the ball before attempting this movement. Often considered an abdominal exercise, this movement uses many muscles, including those of the chest, shoulders, upper and lower back, and legs.

PRONE SKIERS WITH STABILITY BALL

Primary Muscles Used: Abdominals, obliques, pectoralis major, deltoids, core musculature.

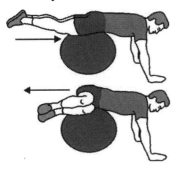

> **Quick Tip:** Performing with only one leg on the ball significantly increases the difficulty of this already challenging exercise.

Exercise Technique: While prone on a stability ball, roll forward until the ball is at the thighs. Arms are extended to the ground under the shoulders and placed about shoulder-width apart with a slight bend at the elbow. Hands are facing forward. The head is neutral. Contract the abs. Flex at the hips and bend at the knees, while moving the bent knees laterally to the side until comfortable. Stop and return to the starting position. Perform the same action on the opposite side. Repeat.

Spotting: The low back should not bow downward. The head should stay neutral and the abs should be contracted.

Comments & Suggestions: This is a very challenging movement. Become proficient at the prone knee tuck before attempting. Start with a very small range of motion and increase slowly as strength and competency improves. One variation is to perform several repetitions on one side and then switch to the other side.

SUPINE LEG SCISSORS WITH STABILITY BALL

Primary Muscles Used: Abdominals (rectus abdominis, internal and external obliques).

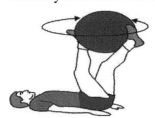

> **Quick Tip:** This exercise becomes more difficult as the extended legs lower toward the ground.

Exercise Technique: Recline supine with a stability ball clasped between the feet. The legs are in the air, extended upward and slightly away from the body. The abs are contracted and the low back pressed into the ground with the arms extended out to the sides. Twirl the ball back and fourth between the feet by rotating the feet around the ball in a semi-circular pattern.

Spotting: The low back should not arch up. Neither the upper body nor the head should come off of the ground during the exercise.

Comments & Suggestions: While often considered an ab exercise, other muscles are also recruited in this exercise, including the hip flexors. This exercise becomes more difficult as the extended legs are lowered closer to the ground. However, a lower leg position also increases the stress on the low back. Discontinue if low back pain occurs.

Free Weights: Pros & Cons

Pro	Con
Inexpensive	Greater risk of injury
Adaptable to all sizes and shapes	Generally more difficult to use
Take up less space	More difficult to isolate single muscle groups
Better activation of stabilizer and synergist muscles	Spotter generally needed for heavy lifts
Not limited to a fixed ROM	Requires greater coordination and skill
Less regular maintenance required	"Fear factor"

Machines: Pros & Cons

Pro	Con
Generally safer to use	Usually expensive
Generally easy to use	Generally uses a fixed ROM
Usually easier to isolate individual muscles	Generally heavy and bulky
Accommodating resistance	Some people may not fit in the machine
Easy to change resistances	More maintenance needed

Chapter 10

HOW HARD ARE PEOPLE EXERCISING?

This chapter deals with some of the various methods that personal trainers may use to determine exercise intensity. Trainers need to understand this because it helps them prescribe a better exercise program for clients.

VO$_2$ Max Test

It is possible to determine how hard you are exercising by measuring how well your cells are using oxygen during exercise. This gives rise to what is called a VO$_2$ test, where "V" stands for "volume" and "O$_2$" is the chemical symbol for the oxygen that we breathe. Stated another way, VO$_2$ is the volume of oxygen that is inhaled minus the volume of oxygen that is exhaled. Typically, the test occurs while a person is exercising on a treadmill or bicycle. An instrument called a spirometer is placed in the person's mouth and the nose is clamped off. The spirometer measures the volume of air that is breathed in and exhaled out by the lungs. As a person exercises, he or she breathes in more oxygen than at rest. As the intensity of exercise is increased, the individual will use even more oxygen in order to supply the body with the energy that it needs to keep pace with the test. At some time during the test, however, a point is reached at which the intensity of exercise becomes too difficult for the body to continue. When this occurs, the person is exercising at maximum capacity and has reached what is called **VO$_2$ max.**

VO$_2$ max is the maximum volume of oxygen that can be taken into the body and used to make energy. Essentially, when you are at VO2max, you are working out as hard as you can aerobically. Studies show that an average VO$_2$ max for most people is around 30–40 mL O$_2$/kg BW/min, where "mL" stands for milliliters, "kg BW" is kilograms of body weight, and "min" means "minute." If you were reading this aloud to somebody, you would say, "30 to 40 milliliters of oxygen per kilogram of body weight per minute." A kilogram is equal to 2.2 pounds. Essentially, this means that when most people are exercising at their maximum, every kilogram (2.2 pounds) of body weight is using somewhere between 30 and 40 milliliters of oxygen per minute. People who work out at a high level on a regular basis can have a VO$_2$ max of above 50 mL O$_2$/kg BW/min.

Once VO2max is known, percentages of this can be calculated. People stay within certain ranges when working out to foster the metabolic changes desired. For generally healthy people, 60–80% VO2 max is usually recommended to support cardiovascular improvements.[25] It is important to note that VO$_2$ max is not just a measure of how well the lungs can take in oxygen. Rather, VO$_2$ max is the result of many body systems all working together for a common goal—energy production. VO$_2$ max involves the heart, lungs, red blood cells, arteries, veins, capillaries, and even the size and number of mitochondria in the exercising muscles.

While typically measured in the lab, one field test that trainers might use to estimate VO$_2$ max was developed by Dr. Kenneth Cooper, the founder of the modern aerobic exercise movement. In this equation, the person runs as far as possible in 12 minutes. The distance covered is converted to meters and the result is entered into this equation:

$$VO_2max = \frac{D_{12} - 505}{45}$$

In this equation, D_{12} is the distance (in meters) that a person runs in 12 minutes. This is subtracted from 505 and the result divided by 45. It should be noted that most clients—especially novices—cannot run for 12 minutes. Because of this, fitness trainers typically prescribe percentages of estimated aerobic ability based on a percentage of the client's estimated maximum heart rate. We will discuss this next.

Factors That Can Influence VO_2 max

Age	VO_2 max decreases as we age. Exercise can slow this decline.
Altitude	Higher altitudes have less oxygen.
Gender	Men tend to have a higher VO_2 max than women. This is not always the case, and exercise can influence this.
Genetics	Genetics plays a big role in VO_2 max. Exercise can increase VO_2 max by about 20% in an untrained person.
Muscles	The muscle's ability to use oxygen.
Heart	The heart's ability to pump blood.
Lungs	The ability of the lungs to absorb oxygen.
Blood	The ability of the blood to distribute oxygen to the body's tissues.

Using Heart Rate

Because heart rate generally increases when we exercise, we can use heart rate to estimate the difficulty of exercise. Let us now discuss the two most popular methods used to measure exercise intensity and then follow our discussion by reviewing other methods with which fitness professionals should be familiar.

Percent of Maximum Heart Rate

The foundation of this method is the equation 220 − Age. By subtracting a person's age from the number 220, you can estimate the maximum number of times his or her heart will beat in 1 minute. For example, if you are 30 years old, 220 − 30 = 190 bpm. Essentially, this number means that, in theory, the heart of a 30-year-old person will be able to beat for no more than 190 bpm if he or she exercises at maximum capacity. You would probably never have anyone exercise at 100% of his or her maximum, so after this number is determined, you calculate percentages of estimated maximal heart rate to arrive at what is sometimes called a **target heart rate training zone,** or THR for short.

Normally, we calculate two percentages and have people stay within that range. For example, you might calculate 60% and 80% of maximum heart rate. When the person becomes fatigued, the pace is reduced until heart rate is closer to the lower level; when he or she feels better again, exercise intensity is increased to the upper end of the range. This is somewhat akin to interval training.

Target Heart Rate Example

Let us use an example to see how this method works. Suppose you are working with a healthy, 45-year-old female. You want this client to exercise at an intensity of 60–75% of the maximum. Here is how to calculate these numbers:

Step 1: 220 – 45 = 175 bpm. (This is the estimated maximum heart rate)

Step 2: 175 x 0.60 = 105bpm   and   175 x 0.75 = 131 bpm

Your calculations are 105 bpm to 174 bpm. Remember, when converting from a percentage to a decimal, all that you have to do is move the decimal point two places to the left. Thus, in this example, 60% = 0.60 and 75% is 0.75.

It is important to remember that the determination of maximal heart rate using the 220 – Age equation is only an estimation. Research shows that actual maximal heart rate may be as much as 10–12 heart beats above or below what is calculated using this equation.[1] Nevertheless, the equation is frequently used because it is easy and convenient. Moreover, it is safer than exercising people to their maximum abilities and then calculating the THR. Many treadmills and other cardiovascular machines also use this equation when estimating heart rate. For example, treadmills typically have programs called "fat burn" and *"cardio."* When you select one of these programs, you are prompted to enter your age. The machine then typically uses the 220 – Age equation to estimate maximum heart rate. Usually, the "fat burn zone" is set at about 60% of maximum heart rate while the "cardiovascular zone" is at 80–85%.

When using this equation with generally healthy individuals, it is usually stated that aerobic benefits occur at 70–85% of one's maximum heart rate.[1] That said, this range may be too intense for some sedentary people to handle. This often causes confusion on the part of trainers who want a cut-and-dry answer to the question, "What percentage range is best?" In reality, there is no perfect answer. As a personal trainer, you must look at the whole person when determining an effective and safe target heart rate range. You will look at age, health issues, past experience with exercise, likes, dislikes, current and past injuries, and goals and blend these together as effectively as possible to develop a target heart rate that is appropriate for each individual person.

Does a Baby's Heart Beat 220 Times a Minute?

People often wonder where the 220 – Age formula originated. Since maximum HR is said to decline one beat per year from a supposed maximum of 220, does this mean that a baby's maximum rate is 220 beats per minute? Of course not. The 220 – Age equation was invented because it seemed to best fit the data that scientists were seeing in their research. In other words, after looking at the numbers, it appeared as though maximum heart rate could be predicted by subtracting a person's age from 220. However, this research has been criticized by others who highlight the lack of original research that specifically examined the validity of the 220 – Age equation.[159] In other words, few studies exist that have actually tested whether the 220 – Age equation accurately predicts maximum heart rate. One of the criticisms against using this equation is that it might overestimate or underestimate one's true maximum heart rate by as much 10–12 bpm according to some reports.[1] Fitness professionals should be aware of this when they use this equation as their sole basis for prescribing an exercise target heart rate. In my opinion, the equation is used best when it coupled with the other methods outlined in this chapter.

The 206.9 – (0.67 x Age) Equation

Because of the problems associated with the 220 – Age formula, several variations have cropped up over the years. One such alternative is the equation 206.9 – (0.67 x Age). This equation is deemed more accurate than most similar alternatives.[189] To use this equation, first do the work inside the parentheses first and then subtract that answer from 206.9. So if you are 45 years old, your maximum heart rate is calculated in this way: Multiply 0.67 x 45 to obtain the number 30.15. Then, subtract 206.9 – 30.15 to obtain the number 176.75, which can be rounded up to 177 bpm. From here, trainers can multiply this number by any percentages of max heart rate that they desire. For more on this equation, how to do the math, and how it stacks up against the 220 – Age formula, see my post, "Is 220-Age The Best Heart Rate Equation?," available at www.Joe-Cannon.com.

Karvonen Heart Rate Formula

In the 1950s, Dr. M. J. Karvonen developed the Karvonen heart rate formula, which is usually considered a more accurate reflection of a person's aerobic stress during exercise and, as such, has been deemed superior to other max heart rate formulas. To use this formula you must first know a person's age and resting heart rate. When you know age and RHR, using the formula is pretty easy and has four steps. They are:

Karvonen Heart Rate Steps

Step 1:	220 – Age
Step 2:	Subtract resting heart rate from step 1
Step 3:	Multiply result of step 2 by percentages you wish to calculate
Step 4:	Add resting heart rate to results of step 3

Note. To improve accuracy, some replace "220 – Age" from step 1 with 206.9 – (0.67 x Age).

The other name for the Karvonen formula is the **heart rate reserve method**. The heart rate reserve is simply the difference between maximal heart rate and resting heart rate. For example, if your maximum heart rate is 180 bpm and your resting heart rate is 60 bpm, your heart rate reserve is 180 – 60 = 120 bpm. The heart rate reserve is being calculated in step #2 of the formula above.

Some may wonder why we should calculate heart rate reserve when determining target heart rate ranges. Think of it this way: simply taking percentages of maximal heart rate (220 – Age, for example) does not take into consideration resting heart rate. The heart rate reserve is the number of heart beats per minute that the heart can *increase* during exercise. In other words, it is your reserve heart beats. Your heart rate does not increase from 0 when you exercise, but increases from its resting rate (RHR). Thus, by subtracting your resting heart rate, you get a better picture of what your heart can do.

Another interesting thing about the heart rate reserve is that, as fitness improves, resting heart rate tends to decrease. This means that the number of reserve heart beats *increases* because the difference between maximal and resting heart rate grows larger. For example, if you were 30 years old and your RHR was 60 bpm, then your heart rate reserve is (220 – 30) – 60 = 130 bpm. After 6 months of working out, your RHR might decrease to 50 bpm. This means that your heart rate reserve is now (220 – 30) – 50 = 140 bpm. You gained an extra 10 bpm that your heart can now increase during exercise.

Let us now illustrate how to use the Karvonen formula with an example. Suppose you want to use the formula to calculate a target heart rate range for a 45-year-old healthy man who has a resting heart rate of 60 bpm. You believe that an intensity of 60–80% of his Karvonen max is enough to sufficiently tax his cardiovascular system safely.

Step 1: 220 – 45 = 175 bpm

Step 2: 175 – 60 = 115 bpm

Step 3: 115 x 60% = 69 bpm   and   115 x 80% = 92 bpm

Step 4: 69 + 60= $\boxed{129 \text{ bpm}}$ and   92 + 60 = $\boxed{152 \text{ bpm}}$

Your answer is 129 bpm–152 bpm. Therefore, you instruct the person to maintain a heart rate of between 129 bpm and 152 bpm, which corresponds to 60–80% of his Karvonen HR max.

The Karvonen formula is usually said to be a more accurate reflection of a person's true aerobic ability. The reason for this is that it closely approximates a person's percent of VO_2 max, the "gold standard" of aerobic conditioning tests. In other words, if a person is working out at 60% of his or her Karvonen HR max, the individual is also close to 60% of his or her VO_2 max. For most healthy people, an intensity of 60–80% of the Karvonen max is sufficient to obtain cardiovascular benefits when working out.[25]

It is important to remember that aerobic improvements can be achieved over a wide range of exercise intensities. Thus, the notion that everybody should work out at 60–80% Karvonen max (or 60–80% HR max) is not engraved in stone. People sometimes get hung up on these numbers and take them as gospel. In reality, they are just guidelines toward which generally healthy people may strive. As a fitness professional, you will likely run into clients who are so deconditioned that a few minutes on a treadmill at a low intensity wipes them out—I have met these people. Because personal training is *personal*, my advice is to look at the health history and PAR–Q forms and talk to the individual about his or her current fitness level. Then, take an educated guess about what you feel is appropriate—and safe—for them at this point in time. I feel that this is a better way to start than adhering to rigid guidelines that do not consider people as individuals.

Exercise Intensities for Generally Healthy People

VO$_2$max	60–80%
Percent of Heart Rate Reserve (Karvonen Formula)	60–80%
Percent of Maximum HR	70–85%

Heart Rate and Blood Pressure Drugs: A Cautionary Tale

One night while working at a health club, I encountered an older man who was a new member. My job at the time was to give new members fitness tests. The health history form did not show anything that seemed like a red flag, so I proceeded with the tests, one of which was a Three-Minute Step Test, used to gauge aerobic fitness. Before the test, I observed that the man's pulse was 60 bpm. Immediately after the test, his pulse was still 60 bpm. Since his pulse did not change, I knew that something was wrong. Looking over the health history form again, I noticed that I had missed something. Stapled to the back of the form was a note from his doctor instructing me to not let his heart rate go above 100 bpm. This man was on a medication called a **beta-blocker,** a drug used to treat high blood pressure and heart problems. One of the side effects of this medication is that it slows down the resting heart rate. Originally, I assumed that his 60 bpm resting heart rate meant he was fit and healthy, but really it was low because he had a serious medical issue and was taking medication. By overlooking that crucial information, I could have really hurt that man.

Because of that incident, whenever I encounter a person who does not exercise and has a low resting heart rate, I assume that they are taking medication for high blood pressure. I suggest that you do the same until you learn otherwise. Even young people may be taking these types of medications. When you encounter people who are on beta-blockers or other medications that slow resting heart rate, *do not use* the Karvonen formula or other heart rate formulas because they are based on heart rate. The medication will make all of your math useless. In this situation, the RPE Scale or Talk Test are better options. Lastly, always look at the back of health history forms.

Other Ways to Measure Exercise Intensity

Trainers often use target heart rates to gauge how hard people are working out, but there are other methods that I feel are superior. These other methods can be used with just about anybody and come in handy when working with someone who may have health problems.

The Talk Test

The talk test is one of the easiest ways to figure out how hard someone is exercising. Basically, if the person can talk while exercising, then he or she is okay. If the person cannot talk during exercise, then he or she is working out too hard.

Studies show that the point when speech first begins to get difficult corresponds with the **ventilatory threshold.**[26] Ventilation is the act of breathing in air and exhaling CO_2. As a general rule of thumb, as exercise intensity increases, ventilation rate increases because you are breathing in and out more quickly to keep pace with your exercise. However, if the intensity of exercise is increased beyond a certain point (i.e., your threshold), then your breathing increases dramatically. This is called the ventilatory threshold.

If you are working with a client and want to use the Talk Test, just ask the person questions during the workout. Sometimes, people begin to mumble answers. If this happens, ask them to speak up. Mumbling or decreasing the pitch of the voice is a way of compensating and could be an indication that the person is at or close to the ventilatory threshold. The ventilatory threshold usually starts to occur between 50–80% Karvonen Max.[25] However, the fitness level is really what determines when it kicks in, so relying on the Karvonen HR may be misleading. Thus, focus primarily on asking the client questions and listening to how he or she replies. If the person says, "I can't talk and do this at the same time," you know that the workout is too difficult.

> ### Are the Ventilatory and Lactate Thresholds the Same Thing?
>
> Another term that usually gets mentioned when you start reading about ventilatory threshold is lactate threshold, also called the anaerobic threshold. While the ventilatory threshold is the point when you start to breathe harder, the lactate threshold is the point during exercise when you begin to anaerobically produce large amounts of lactate. While they tend to occur at about the same time during exercise, they are not the same thing.

Borg Scale

The Borg Scale, also called ratings of perceived exertion (RPE) scale, is a scale from 0–10 that people can use to indicate how difficult exercise feels to them. A rating of 0 is "nothing at all," while a 10 is "maximum effort."

Rating	Meaning
0	Nothing at all
1	Very weak effort
2	Weak effort
3	Moderately strong or difficult effort
5	Strong or difficult effort
7	Very strong or difficult effort
10	Maximum effort

Where the numbers are missing (for example, between 5 and 7), it is understood that the level of intensity is somewhere in between. For example, in the table, level 6 is missing between levels 5 and 7. This indicates that level 6 is an intensity level between these two points.

The RPE scale is usually advocated for gauging exercise intensity in people with high blood pressure as well as those with other health problems. One drawback to the RPE scale is that people must be familiar with what the numbers mean. In other words, if they do not know what the numbers signify, their designations may not be accurate. I recommend giving new clients the RPE scale on a piece of paper to familiarize them with it.

The scale depicted here is actually a modified version of the original, 6–20 scale, where a rating of 6 was "very light activity" and 20 indicated "maximum effort." One difference between the two versions is that the 6–20 scale can also estimate exercise heart rate. For example, a rating of 6 is 6 x 10, or about 60 bpm. A rating of 20 is 20 x 10, or about 200 bpm. For most people, the 0–10 scale is likely easier to understand.

Metabolic Equivalents (METs)

The displays on some treadmills and other cardiovascular equipment may list METs, which can be a useful tool to use for monitoring exercise intensity. **Metabolic equivalents** are basically a comparison between exercise metabolic rate and resting metabolic rate. More specifically, we know that all humans use approximately 3.5 milliliters of oxygen per kilogram of their body weight per minute. This is **1** MET and is usually abbreviated as 3.5 mL O_2/kg BW/min. This is spoken aloud as "3.5 milliliters of oxygen per kilogram of bodyweight per minute." A kilogram is equal to 2.2 pounds. Thus, if we could remove a 2.2-pound chunk from your body and measure the amount of oxygen it is using when you are resting, we would find that it is burning about 3.5 millimeters of oxygen per minute. If you are thinking that this sounds a lot like VO_2, you are correct—METs and VO_2 are very similar. In fact, 1 MET is actually your resting VO_2, which some also call the basal metabolic rate (BMR).[29]

Other Names for 1 MET

1 MET is also:

> ➢ Resting VO_2
> ➢ Basal metabolic rate (BMR)
> ➢ Amount of calories burned at rest

Since METs and VO_2 are basically the same thing and because 1 MET is 3.5 mL O_2/kg BW/min, we can use the number 3.5 to convert from METs to VO_2 and back again. For example, suppose that you are on a treadmill and the display says that you are exercising at an intensity level of 5 METs. What is your VO_2? Here is how to calculate this:

If 1 MET = 3.5 mL/kg BW/min,

then 5 METs = 5 x 3.5 = $\boxed{17.5 \text{ mL/kg BW/min}}$

Essentially, you just multiply the MET number on the treadmill by 3.5 to get the corresponding VO_2. Take note that this answer of 17.5 mL O2/kg BW/min is based on only 1 kilogram (2.2 lb) of body weight. In other words, in this example, each kilogram (2.2 pounds) of the person's body weight is using 17.5 mL of oxygen per minute. If you wanted to obtain the total body VO_2 at which you are working, multiply the VO_2 by bodyweight. For example, if a person weighs 180 pounds (82 kg), you should multiply 17.5 x 82 kg = 1435 milliliters of oxygen per minute.

Do You Have a Slow Metabolism?

Sometimes people who are overweight talk about how they have a slow or sluggish metabolism. However, according to METs, this may not always be true. Remember that while 1 MET equals 3.5 mL O2/kg BW/min, this is on a per kilogram basis. Body weight plays a role in metabolic rate, so heavier people use more energy at rest than thinner people do. Thus, their metabolism is actually higher.

Now suppose that you know the VO_2 but want to know the MET level at which a person is working. In this instance, divide the VO_2 by 3.5. In the example above, the VO_2 is 17.5 mL O2/kg BW/min. To determine METs at this workload, 17.5 / 5 = 5 METs.

Let us say that you do not care to convert METs to VO_2. You can still use METs to determine how difficult exercise feels. Remember that 1 MET also represents the lowest metabolic rate, BMR. BMR can be thought of as the calories burned while sleeping. Thus, if you work out at 2 METs, that means you are burning calories twice has fast as when you are sleeping. If the treadmill says that you are working out at 10 METs, you are burning calories 10 times faster than while sleeping! In general, moderate activity is defined as 3–6 METs, while vigorous activity is defined as more than 6 METs.[35] Keep in mind that the age, physical limitations, and fitness level of a person also factor into what is easy or difficult. For example, it may be easy for a 30-year-old woman to walk to the neighborhood store but very difficult for someone who is 80 or who has physical disabilities. This makes universally quantifying different activities according to METs difficult. When in doubt, it is wise to use METs along with the RPE scale and/or the Talk Test to get a better picture of the difficulty of exercise for a specific person.

It is important for fitness professionals to have a working understanding of METs because they are used clinically to gauge exercise intensity. It is possible that one day you will encounter a person carrying a note from a physician that stipulates that the patient not exercise more than a certain MET level. If you have access to treadmills or bikes that measure METs, this person can be easily accommodated.

In healthy and unhealthy people, evidence suggests that the risk of dying from all causes decreases as cardiovascular fitness improves.[123, 124, 125] In fact, research finds that, on average, each 1-MET increase in exercise capacity might improve survival by 12% in healthy and non-healthy men.[123] In women, these results appear to be even greater, with every increase of 1 MET improving survival by 17%[125]. However, how much exercise does it take to accomplish this? The Surgeon General recommends that everyone engage in moderate physical activity most days of the week (i.e., at least 4 days), if not every day. Other research suggests that burning 2000 calories per week can significantly improve health. With respect to METs, the following equations can be used to estimate the "target MET level" toward which men and women should strive when working out.[124]

Determining Target MET Level

Gender	Equation
Men	14.7 – (0.11 x Age)
Women	14.7 – (0.13 x Age)

For example, a healthy 40-year-old woman should strive to exercise aerobically at an intensity of 14.7 – (0.13 x 40) = 14.7 – 5.2 = 9.5 METs. If achieving this level is not possible due to health reasons, another goal would be to reach at least 85% of the value calculated by these equations. Some research finds double the rates of death in women whose fitness is less than 85% of that predicted by the female equation.[124] Regardless of the numbers, a great deal of evidence suggests that improved physical fitness can help reduce the risk of death in both men and women, and METs can be a powerful tool to help educate and motivate people to stay healthy. If health reasons prevent the achievement of the target MET level, remember that physical activity in general improves health. In other words, doing anything is better than doing nothing at all.

Chapter 11

FITNESS TESTING

Fitness testing is what personal trainers do to get an idea of a person's overall fitness level. This is usually determined soon after the association between client and trainer begins. There is, of course, no single perfect measure of a person's overall fitness. This is why a variety of tests is usually employed. The most common aspects of fitness are as follows:

1. **Muscular strength:** The ability of a muscle to exert force.
2. **Muscular endurance:** The ability of a muscle to contract repeatedly over time.
3. **Cardiovascular endurance:** The ability of the heart, lungs, and blood vessels to deliver oxygen and nutrients to the exercising muscles and remove waste products.
4. **Flexibility:** The range of motion of a joint.
5. **Body composition:** The amount of muscle and fat present on the body.

Some also add **balance** to this list because as a result of aging, disuse, and various medical conditions, balance detriments may be observed. Baseline fitness values can be compared to other people of the same age and gender to determine where a person ranks. Each of the parameters of fitness can be tested. Some of the most common tests for each aspect of fitness are described below. Keep in mind that these are not the only tests available. Thus, you may have used other tests that are not outlined here.

Muscular Strength Tests

10 RM Test

One way to measure muscular strength is to determine the maximum amount of weight that a person can lift for a certain number of repetitions. This is sometimes referred to as an **RM test**. The letters "RM" stand for "repetition maximum" and represent the most weight that a person can lift for a specific number of repetitions with good lifting technique. For example, a weight that is equal to a person's 10 RM is a weight that can only be lifted 10 times with good lifting form. Usually, tests for upper body and lower body strength are used. Classic examples include the bench press for upper body strength and the leg press for lower body strength. To determine the upper and lower body 10RM for someone, follow these steps:

1. After becoming familiar with the equipment, warm up for 5 to 10 minutes with a low-intensity aerobic activity. One may also incorporate a more activity-specific warm-up like performing a set of low-intensity bench presses or leg presses to warm up the muscles even further.
2. Choose a weight that you believe the client can lift *only* 10 times. Be conservative when choosing and do not overestimate what you think the person can lift. If the person can lift more than 10 repetitions, have him or her rest 2–5 minutes and repeat the test with a heavier weight. For the bench press, increase the weight by 5–10 pounds. For the leg

press, increase by 10–30 pounds. Continue the test until a load that can only be lifted 10 times with good lifting form is determined. Try to do this within 3–5 attempts to reduce DOMS.

Some may choose to determine 1RM or the most weight that a person can lift only one time with good lifting technique. This is sometimes considered the "gold standard" of strength testing.[1] Because it entails lifting a considerable about of weight, some feel that it is controversial because of thoughts that it might carry an increased risk of injury. While such objections may be debatable, this test may not be appropriate for beginners or for those with preexisting medical issues. Those who choose to determine 1RM should remember that 1RM testing is also appropriate for smaller muscle groups. For example, attempting a 1RM lift with a biceps curl or triceps extension may cause damage to the joints surrounding those muscles. Thus, 1RM is usually only recommended for the large upper and lower body muscles. Also, any large muscle group exercise that places a person in a risky position (e.g., unsupported bent over row) is generally not appropriate for 1RM testing.

The fact that different people of the same age and gender can usually lift different amounts of weight is the reason why tables listing various 1RM weights are impractical. However, when maximum weight pushed (1RM) is divided by a person's body weight, it is possible to generate a table that can rank a person's 1RM for various ages. The following are tables for the bench press and leg press—the most frequently used measures of upper and lower body strength

1RM Bench Press Strength Values for Men (1RM/Bodyweight)[1, 5]

Ranking	20-29	30-39	40-49	50-59	>60
90	1.48	1.24	1.10	0.97	0.89
80	1.32	1.12	1.00	0.90	0.82
70	1.22	1.04	0.93	0.84	0.77
60	1.14	0.98	0.88	0.79	0.72
50	1.06	0.93	0.84	0.75	0.68
40	0.99	0.88	0.80	0.71	0.66
30	0.93	0.83	0.76	0.68	0.63
20	0.88	0.78	0.72	0.63	0.57
10	0.80	0.71	0.65	0.57	0.53

Percentile Ranking: 90 = well above average; 70=above average; 50 = average; 30 = below average; 10=well below average

154

1 RM Bench Press Strength Values for Women (1RM/Bodyweight)[1, 5]

Ranking	20-29	30-39	40-49	50-59	>60
90	0.54	0.49	0.46	0.40	0.41
80	0.49	0.45	0.40	0.37	0.38
70	0.42	0.42	0.38	0.35	0.36
60	0.41	0.41	0.37	0.33	0.32
50	0.40	0.38	0.34	0.31	0.30
40	0.37	0.37	0.32	0.28	0.29
30	0.35	0.34	0.30	0.26	0.28
20	0.33	0.32	0.27	0.23	0.26
10	0.30	0.27	0.23	0.19	0.25

Percentile Ranking: 90 = well above average; 70=above average; 50 = average; 30 = below average; 10=well below average

1 RM Leg Press Strength Values for Men (1RM/Bodyweight)[1, 5]

Ranking	20-29	30-39	40-49	50-59	>60
90	2.27	2.07	1.92	1.80	1.73
80	2.13	1.93	1.82	1.71	1.62
70	2.05	1.85	1.74	1.64	1.56
60	1.97	1.77	1.68	1.58	1.49
50	1.91	1.71	1.62	1.52	1.43
40	1.83	1.65	1.57	1.46	1.38
30	1.74	1.59	1.51	1.69	1.30
20	1.63	1.52	1.44	1.32	1.25
10	1.51	1.43	1.35	1.22	1.16

Percentile Ranking: 90 = well above average; 70=above average; 50 = average; 30 = below average; 10=well below average

1 RM Leg Press Strength Values for Women' (1RM/Bodyweight)[5]

Ranking	20-29	30-39	40-49	50-59	>60
90	2.05	1.73	1.63	1.51	1.40
80	1.66	1.50	1.46	1.30	1.25
70	1.42	1.47	1.35	1.24	1.18
60	1.36	1.32	1.26	1.18	1.15
50	1.32	1.26	1.19	1.09	1.08
40	1.25	1.21	1.12	1.03	1.04
30	1.23	1.16	1.06	0.95	0.98
20	1.13	1.09	0.94	0.86	0.94
10	1.02	0.94	0.76	0.75	0.84

Percentile Ranking: 90 = well above average; 70=above average; 50 = average; 30 = below average; 10=well below average

For example, suppose a 30-year-old man who weighs 185 pounds had a 1RM of 350 pounds on the leg press. Doing the math, this equals 350 / 185 = 1.89. According to this number, the person is in the 70th percentile for his age and gender for the leg press.

For those who do not want to directly determine 1RM, it is possible to estimate this value with the use of lighter loads and equations. One such equation used to estimate 1RM is the following:[6]

$$1RM = [(\text{number of repetitions} / 30) + 1] \times \text{weight lifted}$$

For example, suppose that a person can lift 150 pounds 10 times. According to the equation, 1RM = [(10 repetitions / 30) +1] x 150 pounds = 200 pounds. Thus, her 1RM is 200 pounds.

It should be stressed that the number determined using this equation (and other equations not mentioned) is only an estimation and may not perfectly reflect a person's true 1 RM. Because of this, some choose to determine 1RM directly. Before doing so, however, people should weigh the risks and benefits of directly determining 1RM before attempting to do so.

Grip Strength Test

This test requires the use of a device called a **dynamometer**. Usually, the dynamometer is held in the hand and squeezed as hard as possible. This test measures isometric hand strength, which is taken as an indicator of overall body strength. While relatively easy to do, the grip strength test may not accurately reflect real life strength. In other words, weak grip strength may not correspond to weak overall strength.

Muscular Endurance Tests

Push-Up Test

In this test, we record the maximum number of good-form push-ups that can be performed. The male client assumes a normal push-up stance, while some females may choose to use a modified bent-knee version. It is important to remember that for some individuals, especially seniors and those with weak upper body strength, push-ups are very difficult to perform. Because of this, the push-up test may end up being a measure of *muscle strength* and not muscular endurance. In addition, the push-up test may be inappropriate for people who have injuries to the shoulder, elbow, wrist, neck, or low back.

Push-Up Test Percentile Rankings for Men[1]

Ranking	20-29	30-39	40-49	50-59	60-69
90	41	32	25	24	24
80	34	27	21	17	16
70	30	24	19	14	11
60	27	21	16	11	10
50	24	19	13	10	9
40	21	16	12	9	7
30	18	14	10	7	6
20	16	11	8	5	4
10	11	8	5	4	2

Percentile Ranking: 90 = well above average; 70=above average; 50 = average; 30 = below average; 10=well below average

Push-Up Test Percentile Rankings for Women[1]

Ranking	20-29	30-39	40-49	50-59	60-69	>70
90	31	27	25	19	18	24
80	27	22	21	17	15	17
70	21	20	17	13	13	11
60	19	17	16	12	11	9
50	18	16	14	11	9	7
40	14	13	11	9	6	2
30	13	10	10	6	4	0
20	10	7	8	3	0	0
10	6	1	4	0	0	0

Percentile Ranking: 90 = well above average; 70=above average; 50 = average; 30 = below average; 10=well below average

Bench Press Test

This test, popularized by the YMCA (hence its alternate name, YMCA Bench Press Test) is similar to the timed push-up test described previously. Men use an 80-pound barbell and women use a 35-pound barbell.[4] This test measures the number of repetitions a barbell can be lifted at a cadence of 30 lifts per minute while reclined on a flat bench.[4] The speed of the lift is set with the use of a metronome. The test is terminated when the person cannot keep up with the metronome's cadence.

YMCA Bench Press Percentile Rankings by Age[3, 5]

Age	18-25		26-35		36-45		46-55		56-65		Over 65	
Ranking	M	F	M	F	M	F	M	F	M	F	M	F
90	44	42	41	40	36	33	28	29	24	24	20	18
80	37	34	33	32	29	28	22	22	20	20	14	14
70	33	28	29	28	25	24	20	18	14	14	10	10
60	29	25	26	24	22	21	16	14	12	12	10	8
50	26	21	22	21	20	17	13	12	10	9	8	6
40	22	18	20	17	17	14	11	9	8	6	6	4
30	20	16	17	14	14	12	9	7	5	5	4	3
20	16	12	13	12	10	8	6	5	3	3	2	1
10	10	6	9	6	6	4	2	1	1	1	1	0

Percentile Ranking: 90 = well above average; 70=above average; 50 = average; 30 = below average; 10=well below average

Another way to gauge muscular endurance is to have the person complete a series of 7 exercises for upper and lower body. This method has the advantage of determining muscular endurance over a wide range of muscle groups and, as such, may be a better predictor of total body muscular endurance. For each exercise, the person lifts a percentage of his or her body weight.[3] The maximum goal for each exercise should be 15 repetitions. Thus, a maximum score for all seven exercises is 7 x 15 = 105 total repetitions lifted. The following table lists the exercises to use in this battery of tests along with the corresponding percentage of body weight that each station should include.

Muscle Endurance Battery of Exercises[3]

Percent of Body Weight To Be Lifted

Exercise	Men	Women	Repetitions performed (max=15)
Bench press	0.66	0.50	
Lat pull down	0.66	0.50	
Leg extension	0.50	0.50	
Leg curl	0.33	0.33	
Triceps extension	0.33	0.33	
Biceps curl	0.33	0.25	
Bent-knee sit-up	Not applicable	Not applicable	
		Total # of Repetitions (max=105)	Total =

For example, using the values from the table, if a man weighs 150 pounds and is performing a bench press, he should lift 150 pounds x 0.66 = 99 pounds. If he is performing the leg curl, he should lift 150 x 0.33 = 49.5 pounds. He should try to complete a maximum of 15 repetitions on each exercise test. No percentage of body weight is associated with sit-ups. The maximum number of repetitions that should be attempted for all tests combined is 105. Make sure that all repetitions are completed with good lifting technique to avoid overstraining or injury. Use the following categories when scoring this test:[3]

Total Repetitions Completed		Meaning
91–105 repetitions	=	Excellent
77–90 repetitions	=	Very good
63–76 repetitions	=	Good
49–62 repetitions	=	Fair
35–48 repetitions	=	Poor
Less than 35 repetitions	=	Very poor

Timed Sit-Up Test

In this test, the person is supine on a padded mat with arms crossed over the chest (touching the shoulders) and knees bent in the usual sit-up position. When the test begins, the person curls up until his or her torso is perpendicular to the floor. Immediately thereafter, the person lowers his or her torso until the shoulder blades are on the mat. The person repeats this as many times as possible in 1 minute. Those who cannot complete 1 minute of continuous abdominal contractions are allowed to rest during the test. However, resting will not affect the time limit of the test. The sit-up test may not be appropriate for individuals who have low back or neck issues, osteoporosis, large abdominal girths, who cannot get up from the floor independently.

Sit-Up Test (YMCA Test) Percentile Rank by Age/Gender[5]

Age	18-25		26-35		36-45		46-55		56-65		Over 65	
Ranking	M	F	M	F	M	F	M	F	M	F	M	F
90	77	68	62	54	60	54	61	48	56	44	50	34
80	66	61	56	46	52	44	53	40	49	38	40	32
70	57	57	52	41	45	38	51	16	46	32	35	29
60	52	51	44	37	43	35	44	33	41	27	31	26
50	46	44	38	34	36	31	39	31	36	24	27	22
40	41	38	36	32	32	28	33	28	32	22	24	20
30	37	34	33	28	29	23	29	25	28	18	22	16
20	33	32	30	24	25	20	24	21	24	12	19	16
10	27	25	21	20	21	16	16	13	20	8	12	11

Percentile Ranking: 90 = well above average; 70=above average; 50 = average; 30 = below average; 10=well below average9

Curl-Up Test

Because sit-ups involve the hip flexor muscles, some favor a modified version that utilizes crunches or partial abdominal curls. This test has two variations. One form of the test has the person complete as many crunches as possible in 1 minute. In this respect, the test is very similar to the timed sit-up test described previously. The other version requires the use of a metronome set to 40 beats per minute (which should allow 20 curl-ups per minute). The person, lying supine on a mat with the arms by the sides, curls his or her torso up until the shoulder blades are off of the floor and then returns to the starting point while keeping pace with the metronome. This continues for as many repetitions as can be completed up to a maximum of 75 repetitions. Like the sit-up test, the curl-up test may not be appropriate for those with osteoporosis, neck problems, older individuals, or those who cannot get up from the floor.

Partial Curl-Up Percentile Rankings[1]

Age	20 - 29		30 - 39		40 - 49		50 - 59		60 - 69	
Ranking	M	F	M	F	M	F	M	F	M	F
90	75	70	75	55	75	50	74	48	53	50
80	56	45	69	43	75	42	60	30	33	30
70	41	37	46	34	67	33	45	23	26	24
60	31	32	36	28	51	28	35	16	19	19
50	27	27	31	21	39	25	27	9	16	13
40	24	21	26	15	31	20	23	2	9	9
30	20	17	19	12	26	14	19	0	6	3
20	13	12	13	0	21	5	13	0	0	0
10	4	5	0	0	13	0	0	0	0	0

Percentile Ranking: 90= well above average; 70=above average; 50= average; 30= below average; 10=well below average

Cardiovascular Endurance Tests

Cardiovascular endurance refers to the ability of the heart, lungs, and blood vessels to deliver adequate oxygen and nutrients to the exercising muscles while at the same time removing waste products that build up and hinder exercise performance. Looking at the big picture, two different paths can be taken to determine cardiovascular (CV) fitness: maximal exercise testing and submaximal exercise testing. **Maximal exercise testing** has a higher degree of accuracy, but it also carries a greater risk of injury (e.g., heart attack). Because of the risks involved, maximal exercise testing should only be performed in the presence of a physician. **Submaximal exercise testing** is how fitness professionals usually determine CV endurance. Here, people are exercised at lower intensities. The information obtained from the test can then be entered into an equation to estimate CV fitness. Cardiovascular endurance is different than muscular endurance, which was described previously. Because of this, different tests are used for each. The following are some of the most common submaximal CV endurance tests used by fitness professionals.

Rockport Walking Test

This test involves having a person walk one mile as fast as possible. The pulse is then taken for one minute immediately after exercise and is entered into an equation to determine CV fitness. Because only fast walking is required, this test is expected to carry a lower risk of injury than tests that involve running. The equation used to determine CV fitness for the Rockport walking test is:[3]

132.853 – (0.0769 x Weight) – (0.3877 x Age) + (6.315 x Gender) – (3.2649 x Time) – (0.1565 x Heart Rate)

For gender, use "1" for males and "0" for females.

These days, it is not necessary to do the math yourself. Just searching the web for "Free Rockport Walking Test Calculator" will reveal many websites that can calculate it for you. If you use the internet, remember to double check the answer on several websites to make sure that you are getting a valid answer. Some personal trainer software programs may analyze the test results also.

The Rockport walking test has been shown to be effective in men and women ages 20–69.[3] Fitness trainers should keep in mind that what is considered "fast walking" for one person may be very different than for another person. Thus, a 69-year-old man will probably walk more slowly than a 25-year-old female.

The 1.5-Mile Run Test

In this test, the person is instructed to cover a distance of 1.5 miles as quickly as possible. Walking is allowed during the test for those who cannot run the complete distance, although the person should be instructed to complete the distance as fast as he or she can. Stretching and warm-up occur prior to the test. From this test, the VO_2 max of the individual can be estimated from the equation:[3]

$$VO_2 \text{ max} = 88.02 - (0.1656 \text{ x Body Weight in Kilograms}) - (2.76 \text{ x Time}) + (3.716 \text{ x Gender})$$

With respect to gender in the equation, enter either "1" for men or "0" for women. An average VO_2 max for many adults will usually be around 30–40 mL O_2/kg BW/min, while for fit people it is typically above 50 mL O_2/kg BW/min.

Other points about this equation to remember:

1. The person's weight is in kilograms. To convert to kilograms, divide body weight (in pounds) by 2.2

2. The time it takes to cover the 1.5 miles should be in minutes. If the distance was not covered in an exact minute (e.g., 10 minutes exactly), convert the seconds into minutes by dividing the seconds by 60. For example, if it took a person 10 minutes and 20 seconds to complete the 1.5 miles, divide the 20 seconds by 60 = 0.33. Thus, the person completed the distance in 10.33 minutes.

1.5-Mile Run Example

Suppose you are testing a 21-year-old female who weighs 120 pounds. She completes the 1.5-mile run in 9 minutes, 10 seconds. Use the 1.5-mile run equation to estimate her VO_2 max.

Step 1. Convert her weight to kilograms. 120 pounds / 2.2 = 55 kg
Step 2. Convert 9 min 10 seconds to minutes. 10 / 60 = 0.17. Thus, she ran the 1.5-mile distance in 9.17 minutes.
Step 3. She is female, so the conversion factor for the equation is 0.

Let us break the equation down into 3 parts to make it easier:
        Part 1. 88.02 – (0.1656 x 55) 88.02 – (9.1) = 78.9
        Part 2. 78.9 – (2.76 x 9.17) = 78.9 – (25.3) = 53.6
        Part 3. 53.6 + (3.716 x 0) = 53.6 + 0 = 53.6

Answer: Her VO_2 max is about 53.6 mL O_2/kg BW/min.

The 1.5-mile run is a relatively good test of cardiovascular endurance, but keep in mind that there is no total agreement that the ability to run for certain distances equals an accurate indicator of VO$_2$ max.[2] The calculation of VO$_2$ max would be less precise in those who cannot run the complete distance or in those who take rest breaks during the test. The test may also not be appropriate in those who have arthritis or other bone and joint disorders, in those with balance problems, or in the elderly. Another issue to consider with this test is that it typically is performed outside, where help may not be readily available if an accident occurs. Bring your cell phone with you just in case.

12-Minute Walk/Run

This test is similar to the 1.5-mile run but is a little less demanding because walking is allowed. Usually, a flat surface like a walking track is used, although a variation of this test could incorporate a treadmill. If a walking track is used, break the track into different sections (e.g., every tenth of a mile) to better determine the distance covered. Some fitness trackers or apps might also be useful. In this test, the person is instructed to cover as much distance as they can in 12 minutes. This can be accomplished by walking, running, or using some combination of both. Stretching before the test might help reduce injury. The distance covered can be used to estimate VO$_2$ max. The equation used to estimate VO$_2$ max is:

$$VO_2 \text{ max} = (0.0268 \text{ x Distance Covered}) - 11.3$$

The distance in this equation is in meters. Thus, if you are working with miles, you will have to first convert miles to meters before using this equation. One mile equals about 1,600 meters. So, if the person ran/walked 2.5 miles in 12 minutes, this equals: (2 x 1600) + (0.5 x 1600) = 3200 + 800 = 4000 meters.

Treadmill Fit Test

Some treadmills and stationary bikes have a built-in 5-minute "fit test" that can be used to estimate CV fitness. This test requires no math on the part of the fitness professional—the fit test does all of the work! While the fit test cannot diagnose any cardiovascular problems, it does give estimates of VO$_2$ max and also indicates how the person compares with others of similar age and gender (i.e., "excellent," "poor," "fair," or "good").

Flexibility Tests

Flexibility is defined as the ability of a joint to move through a full range of motion (ROM). A joint is defined as anywhere two bones meet (e.g., the knee joint or elbow joint). Different joints have different degrees of ROM. For example, the shoulder joint has the greatest ROM in the body. Flexibility depends on a number of issues, including, but not limited to the inflexibility or tightness of ligaments or tendons, age (flexibility tends to decrease as we age), activity level, posture (poor posture may lead to inflexible joints), and even the amount of body fat that a person has. Some research suggests that women may have greater flexibility in some joints than men.[3] Various methods exist to test flexibility. Fitness professionals should remember that no single test can determine the flexibility of all the joints in the body simultaneously.

Sit and Reach Test

This test is designed to measure hamstring and low back flexibility. Following a brief warm-up of simple stretches, the person sits on the floor with the legs extended but not locked. A yardstick can be placed on the floor between the person's legs and a piece of tape placed on the floor at the 15-inch mark on the yardstick. The person is instructed to slowly reach forward with the arms stretched (hands over each other) as far as possible, to hold for a moment, and then to relax. The trainer should ensure that the knees do not bend and that the person does not compensate by reaching further with one hand during the test. Record the distance. Repeat this test 3 times. The furthest point reached is recorded as the individual's low back and hamstring flexibility.

Some may choose to use a sit-and-reach box to perform this test. When using the sit-and-reach box, the person removes his or her shoes and sits on the floor with the feet against the base of the box and legs straight, about shoulder-width apart. The starting position when using a sit-and-reach box is 26 centimeters, which is called the "zero point." After 3 practice tests, the person should extend the arms as before and slowly reach forward as far as possible. Record the distance. Repeat this test 3 times and record the best distance.

Body Composition Tests

Being overweight is defined as having an excess of body weight for one's height and age. The term **obese** is reserved for those who have a body mass index (BMI) of 30 kg/m^2 or more.[1] "Morbid obesity" is defined as being over 100 pounds overweight or having a BMI of 35–40 or more.[160] Body composition generally refers to the amount of muscle and fat a person has. Body fat can be further broken down into **essential fat** (about 3% in men and 15% in women) and **storage fat** (everything other than essential fat). It is sometimes necessary to measure body composition to get a better idea of an individual's general health and disease risk classification.

Average Body Fat Percentages[2]

	Men	Women
Average	12–15%	22–25%
Obese	Greater than 25%	Greater than 30%

Health Risks Associated with Being Overweight[7]*

Premature death from all causes	Type II diabetes	Breast cancer	Pregnancy-related complications
Heart disease	Colon cancer	Endometrial cancer	Gestational diabetes
High blood pressure	Gall bladder cancer	Sleep apnea	Increased surgical risks
Elevated triglycerides	Prostate cancer	Asthma	Irregular menstrual cycles
Decreased HDL	Kidney cancer	Arthritis	Incontinence

*Partial list

Several common measures are available to assess body composition. While some tests are more accurate than others, all have their limitations and drawbacks. Thus, there is no "perfect" test for everybody. The trick is to choose a test that is reasonably accurate and easy to duplicate over time. The following are the more common types of body composition tests of which fitness trainers should be aware.

Body Weight Scales

Many individuals use household scales to estimate body weight. However, the scale only provides one raw number—total body weight. On the downside, scales do not distinguish between fat mass and muscle mass. For example, the scale may not show the full picture for a person who is gaining muscle while losing fat. Scales can, however, be a valuable tool for keeping track of body weight and for tracking weight-loss efforts.

Body Typing

Body typing attempts to classify people into one of three types: ectomorph, mesomorph, or endomorph. The **ectomorph** is said to be thin and have a hard time gaining weight. **Endomorphs** are said to have a hard time losing weight. **Mesomorphs** are defined as having a muscular build and narrow waist. Problems with this type of analysis include the fact that it does not consider percentage of body fat and not everybody fits into one of these three classifications. Also, in theory, classifying according to body type may provide people with a "crutch" that prevents them from pursuing their goals wholeheartedly.

Height-Weight Tables

Height-weight tables determine body composition based on gender and the size of a person's frame. Like scales, height-weight tables do not assess the amount of body fat that a person has. Rather, they compare people to an "average" individual. Problems abound when using only these tables for body composition analysis. For example, many professional athletes are considered overweight when assessed with height-weight tables.[8] Because of error and because alternative superior methods exist, the fitness professional should not rely solely on height-weight tables to determine body composition.

Body Mass Index

The body mass index (BMI) is a number that compares how tall a person is to how much they weigh. It is really more of a general health test than a body fat test. It is easy to determine and only requires a scale and tape measure. The BMI is usually calculated from the equation:

$$BMI = \text{Weight (in kilograms)} / \text{Height (in meters}^2)$$

That is, the BMI is the weight of a person (in kilograms) divided by the person's height (in meters squared). The answer is written using the units kg/m^2. While calculating BMI oneself is usually not necessary anymore thanks to various websites and apps, let us do an example to understand the way that the equation works. Suppose a person weighs 200 pounds and is 6 feet tall. His BMI is calculated as follows:

1. Convert pounds to kilograms. Since there are 2.2 pounds in a kilogram, 200 lb / 2.2 = 91 kg.

2. Convert the person's height to meters squared (m²). Since the person is 6 feet tall and since there are 3.28 feet in a meter, the person is 1.8 meters tall (6 / 3.28). Now, square this number (that is, 1.8 meters x 1.8 meters) to get 3.24m².

3. The person's BMI is 91 kg / 3.24 m² = $\boxed{28.0 \text{ kg/m}^2}$

Another BMI equation that does not rely on the metric system is:

$$BMI = 703 \text{ (Weight in pounds / Height}^2 \text{ in inches)}$$

Even though BMI does not directly measure body fat, in general, the higher the number, the more obesity-related health problems a person tends to have, especially as BMI increases over 25 kg/m².[2] For example, on average, a person with a BMI of 18–25 uses about $4000 annually in health care costs, while those whose BMI is over 40 use about $8000 annually.[161] According to current guidelines, a BMI of 25–29 kg/m² is classified as "overweight" and a BMI of over 30 kg/m² is considered "obese."

One limitation of BMI is that it does not tell the difference between fat and muscle. As such, the BMI scale classifies many professional athletes as "obese." Two people of the same height and weight have the same BMI, yet one person may have 10% body fat while another has 35%. In addition, there is a ± 5% error when determining body fatness from BMI.[1,2] While BMI is a valuable tool, this measure alone does not portray the full picture of a person's health, especially in those who work out. When in doubt, combine the BMI with other measurements to get a clearer picture of a client's health profile.

Body Mass Index

BMI	Meaning
18.5–24.9	Healthy weight
25–29.9	Overweight
> 30	Obese
30–34.9	Class I obesity
35–39.9	Class II obesity
40–49.9	Class III obesity
50–59.9	Super obese
> 60	Super, super obese

Circumference Measurements

The advantage of circumference (girth) measurements is that they are quick and easy and only require a tape measure. While this information can be plugged into equations to estimate body composition, it is more likely that data will be used to help the trainer and client follow changes in girth over time. For those working with very overweight individuals, this method offers a way to track changes while at the same time not making the client feel overly self-conscious. For a more complete picture of body composition, however, combine it with another method (e.g., BIA) if possible.

Usually, measurements of upper limb circumferences are taken in the straightened, un-flexed position. This will provide information on the limb's resting girth. Additionally, some may take measurements of limbs when they are flexed in order to obtain information about how big a muscle is initially and how much it develops over time. Normally, only the right limbs are measured when calculating body composition. If possible, remove excess clothing, as this may lead to inaccurate results. Also, a second person may be needed to properly position the measuring tape (especially around the abdomen and hips). When working with very obese people, remember that the measuring tape may not be long enough to fully encircle abdominal girth. Those wanting to avoid embarrassing situations may wish to not measure this area in very overweight individuals.

Circumference Measurements[3]

Area	Location of Measurement
Neck	At Adam's apple.
Shoulder	At maximum bulges of deltoid muscles. Record after normal expiration.
Chest	Just above the nipple line. Take measurement after normal expiration.
Waist	At the narrowest part of the waist, which is usually above the belly button. Take measurement after normal expiration.
Abdominal	At belly button or at the point of greatest abdominal protuberance.
Hip	At the maximum protuberance of the buttocks.
Thigh	Largest circumference of thigh, close to buttocks.
Calf	At thickest part of calf.
Upper Arm (biceps)	At maximum girth of upper arm when arm is relaxed.
Forearm	At maximum girth of forearm when arm is relaxed.

Abdominal Waist Circumference

Those who carry most of their weight around the belly are at elevated risk of obesity related diseases. Research indicates that men who have a waist circumference greater than 40 inches (102 cm) and women whose waist is greater than 35 inches (88 cm) are at higher risk of heart disease, type II diabetes, hypertension, high cholesterol, and other obesity-related issues.[162] Thus, this measurement is important.

The measurement taken is located at the narrowest part of the waist, usually a little bit above the belly button, after a normal exhalation. The waist circumference can be especially useful in those who are deemed "normal" or "overweight" by BMI alone. In other words, if the BMI indicates that a person is "normal," his or her waist girth may still indicate an increased risk for disease.[162] Thus, calculating waist circumference and BMI appear to be better than BMI alone for some people. This may be particularly helpful when dealing with older adults and Asians, in whom waist girth appears to predict disease risk more accurately than BMI.[162] In those whose BMI is over 35, waist circumference usually adds little to the ability to predict overall disease risk.[162]

Some may also calculate the **waist-to-hip ratio** (WHR). The waist-to-hip ratio is also used to estimate the degree of abdominal obesity, which indicates risk for heart disease. As the WHR increases, the risk of obesity-related diseases also increases.[2] A waist-to-hip ratio greater than 0.95 for adult men or 0.86 for adult women indicates greater disease risk.[3] If waist circumference is determined, however, calculating the waist-to-hip circumference is usually not necessary, as it does not appear to offer any advantages to waist girth alone.[162]

Waist-to-Hip Ratio

Male	Female	Health Risk
≤ 0.95	≤ 0.80	Low Risk
0.96–1.0	0.81–0.85	Moderate Risk
≥ 1.0	≥ 0.85	High Risk

Bioelectric Impedance Analysis

Bioelectric impedance analysis (BIA) is very popular in fitness center because it is quick and easy to administer. This method works by passing a low-intensity electric current through the body and measuring its resistance.[1] Muscle is a better conductor of electricity because of its greater water content. Thus, the current travels faster, resulting in a lower body fat percentage reading. When more fat is encountered, the current travels more slowly due to the reduced water content in fat. In this way, BIA provides a quick and relatively accurate estimate of body composition.

BIA devices usually cost about $50 and come in hand-held versions as well as those on which a person stands. Some models also calculate BMI and still others may have an "athlete mode" that, in theory, may provide a greater degree of accuracy for those who exercise on a regular basis. Whichever type is chosen, the accuracy of BIA depends on following several guidelines:

General BIA Guidelines

1. **Do not** eat or drink for at least 4 hours before the test.
2. **Do not** exercise for at least 12 hours before the test.
3. **Do** urinate 30 minutes before the test.
4. **Do not** drink alcohol for at least 48 hours before the test.
5. **Do not** ingest any diuretics (including caffeine) before the test unless prescribed by physician.

The equations used today in commercially available machines are reasonably accurate for most people. However, some machines may be unable to determine body composition in those with very high or very low body fat. For example, an error message may result in some machines if used on people who weigh over 300 pounds. Error messages may likewise occur in bodybuilders or others who have very low body fat percentages.

BIA may be inappropriate for people who have pacemakers or other implantable heart devices, in whom it is possible that the electric current of the BIA device may accidentally set off the pacemaker or defibrillator. Fitness professionals should ask everyone, regardless of age, whether they have a pacemaker or defibrillator. In addition, BIA should not be performed on pregnant women.

Skin Fold Analysis

Skin fold analysis refers to the use of special calipers that essentially pinch people at different parts of the body to determine the amount of body fat that one has. This method is made possible because a relationship exists between the fat just under the skin (subcutaneous fat) and one's total amount of body fat.[2] Thus, one can estimate total body fat by measuring the fat under the skin.

The caliper device measures the thickness of various skin folds. All readings should be taken on the right side of the body.[3] Also, take measurements before exercise, never afterward. The information obtained is plugged into equations to calculate an estimation of body composition. When performed correctly, the skin fold technique may be accurate to about ± 3%, making it very accurate. The operative word, however, is "correctly." This method takes time to learn.

Drawbacks to Skin Fold Testing

1. Total body fat does not just depend on the fat under the skin. Skin fold analysis cannot determine fat around organs.
2. The degree of accuracy depends on the expertise of the person performing the test.
3. Equations for this method are gender-, age-, and race-specific. Thus, using the wrong equation will generate a less accurate result.
4. Some people are not comfortable being pinched by people whom they do not know.
5. This method may not be appropriate for the very overweight.

While skin fold analysis can be accurate, fitness professionals should remember that new clients may not enjoy being pinched by people whom they do not know well. Also, some may not enjoy body fat analysis in general. That is, thin people may enjoy seeing their low percentage of body fat while overweight people may not.

Fitness professionals have probably witnessed the frustration of people who, after dieting and exercising for several weeks, only manage to decrease their body fat by a percentage or two. While this may amount to several pounds of lost fat, seeing a drop of only 1% can be discouraging. To combat this, another option is to simply add up all of the measurements for each site.[16] In other words, record the areas as you normally do and add them up. Then, several weeks or months later, do the same thing again—record the measurements and add them up. In theory, this second result will be smaller if the person has lost body fat. For example:

Site Measured	Measurement (August)*	New Measurement (December)*	Difference (Aug – Dec)
Triceps	11.9	9.7	2.2
Quadriceps	32.5	29.5	3.0
Abs	25.8	22.5	3.3
Suprailiac	14.0	11.0	3.0
Totals	**84.2**	**72.7**	**11.5**

*All measurements in millimeters

In this example, you can see that all the measurements taken in August add up to 84.2 millimeters. When the same sites are measured again in December, the sum is 72.7 mm. This means that the person has lost 11.5 mm overall since August (84.2 - 72.5=11.5). For some clients, this might be a better method than stating that the person lost 1% of their body fat. Because this method requires close contact between persons, trainers using it should only take measurements in the presence of a third party to reduce the risk of touching being misinterpreted and allegations of sexual harassment being made.

Near Infrared Interactance

The estimation of body composition by near infrared interactance (NIR) makes use of a specialized probe that is placed against an area of the body (e.g., the biceps) and that emits infrared light that passes through muscle and fat. Fat and muscle absorb and reflect different frequencies of light, and the NIR machine uses this information along with age and activity level to estimate body composition. While variations of this technique have been used in clinical settings since the 1960s, portable devices that are commercially available have been shown to be less accurate than the skin fold techniques and bioelectric impedance analysis described above. Some research finds that NIR might overestimate body fatness in lean people and underestimate it in overweight people.[162] More study is needed before NIR becomes universally accepted.

Hydrostatic Weighing

Hydrostatic weighing is often called the "gold standard" of body composition analysis because it is one of the most accurate methods and the basis upon which all others are compared. Because of this, hydrostatic weighing is often used in clinical research. The other name for this is "underwater weighing," a phrase derived from the fact that people are completely submerged underwater to determine body composition. Hydrostatic weighing is based on Archimedes' Principle—that is, a body buoyed in water will be forced to the surface by a force equal to the volume of water that it displaces. In other words, fat floats—the more fat a person has, the lighter they will be when weighed underwater. Usually the person is submerged underwater while seated on a scale. The individual then forcibly exhales as much air from the lungs as possible and remains motionless. Measurements of body weight under water and on land are plugged into equations that yield the body fat percentage. For individuals who are uncomfortable with being submerged underwater and for those who are not comfortable being in a bathing suit, this method can be a frightening experience. While accurate, underwater weighing requires special equipment and, as such, is unlikely to be offered in a health club setting.

Air Displacement

Just as hydrostatic weighing measures the displacement of water, body composition can also be determined by measuring the amount of air that a person displaces. The most popular of these types of machines is the Bod Pod®, which measures air displacement when people sit in a special sealed chamber. Clinical studies have been published on the Bod Pod, and many find it to be accurate in numerous groups of people.[10, 11] While body composition can be determined in a matter of minutes using this equipment, it can cost tens of thousands of dollars, putting it out of reach for many health clubs.

Dual Energy X-Ray Absorptiometry

In addition to its more common use—determining bone density—dual energy x-ray absorptiometry (also known as a "DEXA Scan") can also precisely estimate the amount of fat and lean muscle tissue present in the body. Some consider this method to be more accurate than underwater weighing. That said, because it uses low-level radiation, it is usually reserved for hospitals and other clinical research settings.

Estimating Muscle Mass

People sometimes want to know how much muscle is on their bodies. If you know their percentage of body fat, you can estimate this. For example, suppose that someone is 200 pounds and is 20% body fat. 200 x 0.2 = 40 pounds of fat. Subtract this from the total body weight and you get 200 – 40 = 160 pounds of fat-free mass, which we typically refer to as muscle. Remember, this calculation is only an estimate. For example, fat-free mass is not just muscle, but also includes things such as bone, water, hair, and more. Another possible area for error is in measuring percentage of body fat. Many techniques (BIA, skin folds, etc.) are not 100% accurate. Failure to adhere to the guidelines of these methods will ramp up inaccuracy.

Additional Tests

In addition to tests of strength, endurance, and the other areas previously mentioned, it is wise to also measure both resting heart rate and blood pressure. These are important because they may give valuable clues as to the general health of the individual.

Resting Heart Rate

Resting heart rate (RHR) is the number of times a heart beats at rest. We obtain RHR by measuring the pulse, which is the sensation that we can feel as blood is pumped through the blood vessels. While medical professionals usually take note of the strength of the pulse as well as its rhythm, fitness trainers usually just measure the number of beats that the heart makes in a minute because this can reflect one aspect of general physical fitness.

The average resting heart rate of an adult is 60–100 bpm.[5] A resting heart rate above 100 bpm is technically classified as **tachycardia,** and a resting heart rate below 60 bpm is usually called **bradycardia**. These terms are general and, without medical interpretation, do not mean much. In other words, tachycardia could be caused by heart disease, emotional stress, some dietary supplements, or simply running up a flight of stairs. By the same token, bradycardia could be caused by some medications (e.g., beta blockers) as well as long-term regular exercise.

Resting Heart Rate and Overtraining Syndrome

Overtraining syndrome represents a series of related issues that tend to occur when a person spends so much time working out that he or she does not give the body enough time to recover properly. This, in turn, can lead to a decrease in exercise performance. One of the signs of overtraining syndrome is an elevation of resting heart rate. For example, someone with this condition may have a RHR of 85 bpm—even though they work out 3 hours a day, 7 days a week!

While overtraining syndrome is unlikely in the typical person who exercises, it is a real possibility in professional and amateur athletes and "gym rats" alike. The only cure for overtraining syndrome is to drastically cut back on the length and intensity of workouts. It may take a few months for symptoms to subside. Keeping a record of resting heart rate is one of the easiest ways to avoid overtraining syndrome. Other classic signs of this condition include increased infection rate, increase in number of injuries, insomnia, and decreased exercise performance.

When taking a pulse on another person, it is best to do so at the radial pulse, located on the thumb side of the wrist, rather than at the carotid arteries on the sides of the neck. This is because there are pressure receptors in the carotid arteries of the neck and pressing too hard activates these receptors and stimulates a nerve that slows the heart rate.[2] When taking the pulse, use the index and middle fingers to palpate the area; do not use the thumb, as it has its own pulse and this may interfere with your reading.[2] While the best time to obtain RHR is in the morning before people get out of bed, for trainers, having the person sit quietly for 5–10 minutes prior to taking the measurement will usually suffice. People should also refrain from smoking or consuming caffeine for at least 30 minutes prior to the test, as both of these can elevate heart rate. Some weight loss and herbal supplements may also raise HR, so this may need to be considered when evaluating the results.

When taking a pulse, count the first beat as "one," followed by "two," "three," and so on. Do not start with "0," as this will add an extra beat to the count. Some people choose to take the pulse for an entire minute, while others may take it for 30 seconds and then multiply the result by 2 (30 x 2 = 60 seconds). When first learning to take the pulse, do so for a full minute to make sure that you counted correctly. Remember, the shorter the time, the greater the error if you miscount. For example, if you are taking a pulse for 6 seconds and you miss a beat, your answer will be off by 10 beats.

Some research suggests that heart rate may provide information regarding long-term health. For example, one study involved 5,700 apparently healthy men who were given exercise tests and then followed by researchers for 23 years.[15] Decades after the initial tests, researchers noted that some of the men were at increased risk of sudden death. This observation was seen: 1) in men who had a RHR of more than 75 bpm; 2) in men whose heart rate increased by less than 89 bpm during maximal exercise; and 3) in men whose heart rate decreased by less than 25 bpm after exercise was stopped. Since long-term exercise tends to lower RHR, taking note of a new client's RHR may arm fitness trainers with knowledge that can help people avoid health problems down the road.

Factors That Impact Heart Rate

When someone takes a heart rate, whether it is upon waking or at another time, they are in effect taking a "snapshot" of the heart rate at that particular point in time. Heart rate (and blood pressure) changes throughout the day. How it changes can depend on a number of environmental, nutritional, emotional, and pharmacological factors. For example, some ingredients in weight loss products many raise heart rate. Yohimbe and bitter orange (citrus aurantium) are just two examples of ingredients known to do this. Caffeine and smoking can also elevate heart rate. Even walking up a flight of steps can significantly alter heart rate.

Factors That Can Alter Heart Rate and Blood Pressure

Stimulants	Some herbal supplements
Smoking	Emotional stress
Digestion of food	Age
Position of the body	Time of day
Some medications	Exercise or physical exertion

Some medications can affect heart rate. In general, a resting heart rate of 60 bpm or less in people who do not exercise may signify that the person is taking heart or blood pressure medications like beta blockers, which slow resting heart rate. When working with these people, it is better to use either the Talk Test or RPE Scale rather than assigning a target heart rate. Medication usage like this should be a red flag to trainers that significant medical issues exist. In such instances, both client and trainer are best served if a written release from the client's physician is obtained prior to training.

Blood Pressure

Blood pressure is the pressure of the blood exerted on the walls of the blood vessels. As the heart beats, it squeezes blood through the blood vessel system. The pressure of the blood as it is pushed through the blood vessels can be easily measured by listening for sound vibrations called Korotkoff sounds. All that is needed is a stethoscope and a blood pressure cuff (sphygmomanometer). When the blood pressure cuff is wrapped around the upper arm and inflated, it eventually cuts off the blood supply. This usually occurs when the cuff is inflated to a pressure of between 180–220 mm Hg (mm Hg means "millimeters of mercury").

Blood pressure is actually made up of two separate pressures written as a fraction. They are called the **systolic** (pronounced sis-tol-ik) blood pressure and the **diastolic** (pronounced die-is-tol-ik) blood pressure. For example, if your blood pressure is 120/80, 120 is your systolic pressure and 80 is your diastolic pressure. More specifically, the systolic pressure is the blood pressure that results when the heart is contracting to push blood out of the heart. Diastolic pressure is the pressure in the blood vessels when your heart is filling with blood to prepare to contract again.

Blood Pressure Ranges[75]

Normal	Less than 120/80
Prehypertension	120/80–139/89
Hypertension	Greater than 140/90

Personal trainers do not diagnose hypertension—only a physician can diagnose a disease or condition. Fitness trainers can make clients aware of abnormal blood pressure readings so that the individual can take that information to his or her physician for a more in-depth follow up.

Some people believe that 120/80 is "normal," but in the table above, we see that it is not. Less than 120/80 is now considered normal, while a pressure of 120/80 is called **prehypertension**. This term was invented in 2003 in light of research showing that men over 50 years of age had a 90% chance of developing high blood pressure at some point in their lifetimes if they started out with a BP of 120/80.[17] High blood pressure is often called the "silent killer" because it does not have any overt signs or symptoms until it is too late. On prescription pads, physicians will usually abbreviate hypertension as "HTN" or "HBP."

How to Take Blood Pressure

Blood pressure should be measured in a comfortable, seated position with feet on the floor. Ideally, 5 minutes of rest should precede the test to help normalize blood pressure. The person should not smoke for at least 30 minutes before the test. Supinate the arm so that the palm is facing up. The blood pressure cuff should be wrapped around the upper arm at the level of the heart.[1] The arm should be resting on a table or chair. Either the right or left arm can be used. Because blood pressure can vary slightly between the left and right arms, it may be wise to measure both arms and choose the side that gives the higher reading.

While electronic blood pressure monitors are convenient, learning to take the measurement yourself is not overly difficult. Here is how to do it: Place the stethoscope over the brachial artery and inflate the cuff to about 180–220 mm Hg, or about 20 mm above what the person's blood pressure usually is. Slowly let the air out of the cuff, taking note to listen for sounds. The first sound you hear will be the systolic blood pressure. The point where you no longer hear any other sound is the diastolic blood pressure. Record these values as the person's blood pressure. For example, if you heard the first sound at 120 mm Hg and ceased to hear sounds at 80 mm Hg, the person's blood pressure is 120/80 mm Hg.

Steps for Taking Blood Pressure Readings[1]

1. People should not smoke or use caffeine for at least 30 minutes before the test.
2. Have the person sit quietly for about 5 minutes before the test.
3. If the person wears long sleeves that bunch up when rolled up the arm, ask him or her to remove the garment prior to testing if possible.
4. Wrap the blood pressure cuff around the upper arm at the level of the heart.
5. Line up the cuff with the brachial artery.
6. The stethoscope should be placed over the brachial artery, located in front of the elbow at the antecubital space.

7. Inflate the blood pressure cuff to between 180–220 mm Hg, or about 20 mm Hg above what you think the person's systolic blood pressure is.
8. Slowly release the pressure in the cuff and listen for sounds.
9. The first sound you hear is the systolic BP. Note the pressure when you no longer hear any sounds. This is the diastolic BP.

When taking blood pressure, keep in mind to use the correct blood pressure cuff size. A cuff that is too small can overestimate blood pressure, while a cuff that is too big can make blood pressure seem lower than it truly is. To determine this, first measure the arm circumference with a tape measure. Measure the upper arm midway between the elbow and shoulder.[5] If the circumference is 18–24 cm, use the "child" cuff. For circumferences that are 24–32 cm use the standard "adult" size. Finally, for circumferences of 32–42 cm use the "large adult" cuff.[5] Blood pressure cuffs are sold at most medical- and nursing-supply stores.

Possible Sources of Error When Testing Blood Pressures[1]

Wrong size cuff	Room noise	Too much pressure on stethoscope
Inability to hear Korotkoff sounds	Inexperience of person giving test	Holding on to treadmill/bike (if testing during exercise)
Improper stethoscope placement	Clenching fists/arms during test	Deflating cuff too quickly/slowly
Sphygmomometer not calibrated	Stethoscope is used backward	Stethoscope is under BP cuff

While it is unlikely that most trainers will be taking blood pressure during exercise, those who do should remember that the normal response of blood pressure to aerobic exercise is for the systolic blood pressure to increase as exercise intensity is increased. The diastolic BP will either remain unchanged or may decrease very slightly. Failure of the systolic BP to rise as exercise is made harder may be a sign of an emergency. In this case, the heart cannot meet the demands of exercise any longer. Repeat the BP test immediately and if you get the same result, stop the exercise test and call 911.

Types of Blood Pressure Cuffs

The type of blood pressure cuff used mostly in research and clinical settings is the mercury cuff. This is the type that is considered the "gold standard" because it is most accurate and does not need to be recalibrated over time. When inflated, a column of mercury rises in a glass chamber.

Another popular sphygmomanometer is the aneroid type. This blood pressure cuff is easily recognized because, instead of a vertical column of mercury, it has a round dial with a small needle inside. As the cuff is inflated, the needle moves to greater pressures. While popular, this type may need to be recalibrated over time. Occasionally, readings with aneroid blood pressure cuffs should be compared to those obtained with the more accurate mercury-filled versions for confirmation.

Electronic versions of blood pressure cuffs are also available to the public. These machines inflate automatically and take blood pressure with just the touch of a button. While they may have merit in some situations, they are not as accurate as either mercury or aneroid blood pressure cuffs for all individuals and should not be used in place of seeing a physician regularly. Some portable types measure blood pressure around the wrist. This may also lead to additional points of error.

Recognizing Heart Attacks and Strokes

Signs of a Heart Attack[89]

1. **Chest pain or discomfort.** The chest pain or discomfort can last for as little as 3–5 minutes or go away and return later. The pain can be perceived as a squeezing of the chest or just an uncomfortable feeling.
2. **Pain elsewhere on upper body.** Heart attack pain may also be felt in the jaw, stomach, back, or in one or both arms.
3. **Shortness of breath.** This may or may not accompany chest pain.
4. **Other symptoms.** Less common symptoms of a heart attack can be sweating, light-headedness, or nausea and vomiting.

In addition to chest pain or discomfort, according to the American Heart Association, women may be more likely to complain of other symptoms like shortness of breath, nausea and vomiting, or pain in the jaw or back.[89]

Stroke Warning Signs[88]

1. Sudden numbness or weakness in the face, arm or leg—especially limited to one side of the body.
2. Sudden confusion or trouble speaking or understanding.
3. Sudden trouble seeing out of one or both eyes.
4. Sudden trouble walking, dizziness, loss of coordination, or loss of balance.
5. Sudden severe headache with no known cause.

Medical Emergencies

I have personally witnessed people die while in the gym and I know trainers who have lost clients to heart attacks during personal training sessions. Having lectured to tens of thousands of people over the years and having listened to eyewitness accounts, I can tell you that this happens more than you think. Coming face-to-face with a heart attack, stroke, or other medical emergency can be a traumatic experience, and it is normal to be afraid. That said, if we are able to help as personal trainers, I think that we owe it to our fellow human beings to do whatever we can. Even if that means only calling 911, this is better than doing nothing. Personal trainers may be the most qualified people in the gym who are able to render assistance until paramedics arrive. I say this not to scare anyone, but to equip you with this knowledge just in case it happens on your watch. I believe that it should be mandatory for all fitness trainers have a current CPR and AED certification. These are easy to get and are offered at most hospitals, fire stations, YMCAs, and community colleges.

If you work at a gym, please ask the fitness director or owner what procedures are to be followed in the event of a medical emergency. It has been my experience that some health clubs have well-laid-out plans while others do not. Even if the fitness center where you work does not have a plan in place, my hope is that you are able to plant a seed in the minds of those in charge to address this critical part of member safety.

For much more on this very important topic see my blog post, "Gym Emergency Procedures: What Would You Do?," which may be found at www.Joe-Cannon.com. There, I cover in detail, what I believe should be done during what may be your worst day ever as a personal trainer. Please read it.

Chapter 12

GETTING A JOB IN FITNESS

One of the most frequent questions asked by people just starting out is how to go about obtaining a first personal training job. At your first job, you will learn many of the crucial skills that will ultimately shape you as you grow in the field. While knowing the aspect of fitness in which you want to specialize (kids fitness, seniors, etc.) is important, most have no idea where to go when they are first begin. This chapter is included to help give you the advice and tools that you will need to land a job—and make a lasting impression.

Where Will You Work?

Even if your ultimate goal is to go into business for yourself, you will probably start out by working for someone else. For many, this means working in a fitness center. This is actually a pretty good place to start, because gives you the opportunity to familiarize yourself with a wide range of exercise equipment. This information can help you years later if you are asked by future clients to recommend equipment for their homes. You also have the opportunity to learn other aspects of the fitness business, including sales, the front desk, manager responsibilities, and equipment maintenance, to name a few. If you work in a health club, it is in your long-term best interest to expose yourself to as much about the organization as possible. What you learn now will serve you in the future.

Advantages of Working in a Fitness Center

Exposure to wide range of fitness equipment	Interaction with many different types of people	Learning from others
Making business contacts	Potential to move up the corporate ladder	Learning how to deal with various types of people
Management training	Opening and closing procedures	Front desk operations

Many times, getting an interview may be as easy as walking in the front door of a club and asking for either the Fitness Director, GM, or Manager on Duty (MOD). These are the people who generally have the ability to hire or get you an interview. Sometimes you may be asked to complete an application on the spot, while other times they may make you return at a future date for the interview. When in doubt, it is good to be prepared.

When looking for a job, it is a wise to survey several fitness centers before you actually apply for a position. That way, you will know in advance what each has to offer. Also, feel free to apply to several positions at once. This reduces the chances that you will be behind the eight ball, waiting for a single prospective employer to call you back.

Interviewing for a Job

Interviewing for a job can be stressful, but it does not have to be—it is not only *they* who are interviewing you but *you* who are interviewing them! This is your time to ask questions and determine if the position suits your needs. Before the interview, take note of these tips to help you make a lasting impression.

1. **Bring your resume with you.** Your resume does not have to be fancy or have industry-specific experience. On your resume, list your fitness certifications, CPR/AED certifications, college degrees or other educational experience, internships, previous fitness-related experience, fitness-related interests, and any skills that you feel would help the company. If you have competed in the Ironman Triathlon, climbed Mt. Everest, or done anything unique, include this as well. If you are brand new to the industry, do not worry if you do not have much experience. The fact that you present a resume will speak volumes about your character and professionalism. Do not worry if you have never created a resume, either—they are easy to compose. Sample resumes can be found online, and many books show you how to write one as well. Bring your resume to the interview in a padfolio for safe-keeping. Carry it in your left hand so that you can easily shake hands with people. The padfolio should have paper and pencil available for you to take notes during the interview. This is also a place for you to write the questions that you have about the job for which you are interviewing. Write these questions down before the interview. This communicates to employers that you are taking the position seriously.

2. **Dress appropriately for the interview.** Generally, fitness is a casual field, so dressing up in a suit and tie is usually not necessary (unless you are interviewing for a management or GM position, in which case it is). Khakis, casual shoes, and a polo shirt are sufficient for most fitness job interviews. Dressing for the interview says to management that you are a mature person who takes the interview seriously. This elevates you over all others who do not dress up.

3. **After the interview, send a thank-you letter.** A thank-you letter is a common courtesy in business and should be mailed a day or two after the interview. Just a short letter thanking the person for his or her time is all that is needed. Generally, handwritten notes are more personal than emails or those typed on a computer. The letter demonstrates to the employer that you appreciate the time they spent interviewing you. Include your phone number and address to make it easier for the person to reach you. Most people in fitness probably will not send a thank-you note, so this is another excellent way for you to stand out in the eyes of management. Even if you do not get the job that you want, the odds are very good that management will remember your name and, if an opening occurs in the future, you probably will be first on their list to contact.

Interview Questions

During the interview you will be asked questions so that the organization can get to know you better. Here is a list of very common questions that you may be asked during an interview. It is suggested that you review these questions and think about your answers ahead of time.

Possible Interview Questions

1. Why do you want to work for us? (Probably the most common question asked)
2. Where do you see yourself in 5 or 10 years?
3. What do you feel are your strengths?
4. What do you feel are your weaknesses?
5. Why should we hire you for this job?
6. Do you prefer to work alone or as part of a team?
7. Give an example of a difficult situation you have faced and how you resolved it.
8. Why did you leave your most recent job?
9. How would you describe your style of management?
10. What would you say is the biggest difference between us and your previous employer?

Questions You Should Ask during an Interview

A job interview is not just for the employer to ask you questions—it is a time for you to ask questions, too! By asking questions of your potential employer, you send a strong message that you have done your homework about their organization. A good place to start is with the company's website.

Possible Questions to Ask during an Interview

1. How many members does the club currently have?
2. What is the average age of the club's members?
3. With which organizations are the fitness staff certified?
4. What is the fitness philosophy of the health club?
5. What are the duties/responsibilities of the position for which I am interviewing?
6. Are there any skills that you feel are crucial to success in the position?
7. How will my job performance be measured and by whom?
8. Does the club provide any educational incentives to help me advance my knowledge?
9. Is there room for growth within the organization?
10. What are the established procedures to follow in the event of a medical emergency?

This last question, asking about emergency procedures, I feel is particularly important given that accidents—minor and serious—do occur from time to time in health clubs. Having a competent staff makes a manager's job easier. Nowhere is this more important than in an emergency situation. Also, you may be the only one who has ever asked this question, which again sets you apart from the rest of the pack in the eyes of management.

Interview Mistakes

Years ago, I applied for a job in telemarketing. During the interview, I was asked the dreaded question, "Why do you want to work for us?" to which I replied confidently, "Because it is easy!" Needless to say, I did not get the job. Truth be told, the job was easy compared to my last job where I washed dishes in a hot kitchen for so long that the skin flaked off of my hands. The person interviewing me did not care that I left for the interview at 6 am and took two buses in the pouring rain to be on time for the interview. In her mind, all she heard was that I did not take the job seriously. To make sure that your interview goes well, never say that the job is "easy," and follow these additional tips.

Tips for a Great Interview

---

1. Show up on time for the interview.
2. Turn your cell phone off. If your phone rings during the interview do not answer it.
3. Do bring your resume and dress appropriately.
4. Do not talk badly about former employers during the interview.
5. Do maintain eye contact when speaking.
6. Be friendly yet professional during the interview.
7. Do know about the company ahead of time—check their website.
8. Do mirror the demeanor of the interviewer. If he or she is all business, you be all business, too.
9. Do mention your strengths and how they would fit with the organization.
10. Do be enthusiastic about the job for which you are interviewing.

How Much Is the Salary?

At some point during the interview, the salary of the position will probably be addressed by the person doing the hiring. While some feel that it is rude for the interviewee to ask about salary, I do not, especially if the issue is not brought up by the time the interview is almost over.

With respect to fitness trainers, salary is usually composed of an hourly wage plus commissions. The hourly wage will vary but is generally $6–$20 per hour for "floor time"—the time fitness trainers are in the fitness center, helping members, and trying to get clients. Commissions are where fitness trainers usually make most of their money. Generally, personal training and fitness commissions range from 40–65% of the amount paid to the club. For example, if a member pays $50 for a personal training session and the trainer gets a 50% commission, he or she makes $25 for that session. While sessions may last 60 minutes, at many clubs they are only about 30 minutes.

Some health clubs may pay different commission rates based on your education, years of experience, and other factors. This sometimes leads to titles like "Level One Trainer" or "Master Trainer." Clubs generally want to hold onto good personal trainers, and they tend to reward those who continue to sharpen their skills.

Since I first created this book, I have written much more on these topics at Joe-Cannon.com. For those who want to know more, I will direct you to these blog posts for more information:
- "Fitness Job Interview: Steps to Success"
- "Personal Trainer Resume Tips"
- "Certified but Never Train ed Anyone: What To Do"

Chapter 13

QUESTIONS AND ANSWERS

For years, I have received emails from people all over the world who are looking for answers to their fitness questions. Here are some of those questions. I picked these to give trainers an idea of what they may be asked by future clients and by others. They may even be questions that they have themselves.

Q. How can I get clients?

A. I have often said that getting certified is easy and getting clients is the hard part. That said, here are some ideas that may help. **1.** Start a free walking club in your neighborhood. It is a chance for your neighbors to get to know you and become familiar with your other services. **2.** Offer free blood pressure readings at the gym where you work. If you are the only person who knows how to do this, the members assume that you are the smartest trainer. **3.** Help the gym sales people give tours to new members. **4.** Smile at the gym members and learn their names. **5.** Do not hang out with other trainers when inside the gym. Members will not approach you if you are in a group. **6.** Teach a group exercise class, because some of those people may hire you. **7.** Pass business cards out to bridal salons and similar businesses. **8.** Specialize in only certain areas of fitness. This helps you become known as an "expert." **9.** Give T-shirts featuring your business name to current clients. This makes your clients "walking advertisements" for you. **10.** On the back of your business cards, offer a free or discounted service like fitness testing. This helps get people in the door. **11.** Make a website. New clients will want to check you out online first. I show you how to make a website at Joe-Cannon.com. **12.** Give seminars to local businesses. Not only will businesses pay you for this, but some of their employees may become clients. By the time you read this, I may have posted additional ideas on my website, so be sure to look there also.

Q. Is muscle confusion real?

A. The idea behind muscle confusion is that we have to keep the muscles "guessing" with different exercises in order to see improvements in fitness. What is often left out of this idea that the muscles need to be overloaded with more stress than they are used to. In other words, what if we tried to "confuse" the muscles with less intensity? Would they grow then? Probably not. As a muscle grows stronger, requires greater intensities to improve—not necessarily just variations in the types of activities.

While the idea appears to share some things in common with both cross training and periodization, muscle confusion is not a scientific principle. I am not aware of any scientific studies showing that programs that employ "muscle confusion" result in greater fitness, EPOC, or reduced injuries compared to more traditional exercise programs. Since most people who hire personal trainers are beginners, there is no need to try to "confuse" the muscles with different exercises several days a week because everything is new to the novice and will remain that way for several months. Using periodization to improve fitness is scientifically validated. The same cannot be said for muscle confusion.

Q. What precautions should female trainers take before going to the home of a new client?

A. Because of the internet, it is sometimes possible to discover information about the client before meeting with him or her. Checking your area's sex offender registry website may also help. At least one friend should know the location of all client's names and addresses. Trainers should also carry a cell phone with them and call a friend or significant other just prior to entering a client's home, especially if they do not know the person. Most cell phones can be tracked via GPS. They should tell the friend the name and address of the client with whom they are meeting, as well as the start and end times of the session. Call that friend again when the session ends. Some trainers will make a point to mention during the session that they have an appointment immediately after the meeting so that the client knows the trainer is expected elsewhere. The trainer might even let the client see him or herself talking on the phone when the client opens the door. Some women may also carry pepper spray or other personal defense items. Women should be suspicious of people who want to meet at night or in secluded locations. Those who make strange requests may also be called into question. Never feel pressured to meet someone if you do not feel comfortable while talking to that person on the phone. Technically, both men and women should take precautions like these because, unfortunately, the world is not as safe as it used to be.

Q. One of my clients is sexually harassing me. What can I do?

A. You may want to pass the client along to another trainer. You should also discuss the matter with the club's general manager and let him or her take appropriate action against the offending club member. It is also wise to document all occurrences of the harassment, noting the dates and times of the incidents, witnesses, and as many specifics as you can recall. Copies of the incidents should go to the GM, and you should also retain copies for your own records. The gym is obligated to provide a safe environment for its employees, and this includes being free from sexual harassment from the club's members and other staff. The GM should keep you in the loop regarding the action that he or she has taken to deal with the problem. If the harassment continues, you have other legal options that an attorney can provide. The same procedure also applies to men who are sexually harassed.

Q. My client feels a burning sensation in their calves when they walk. It stops after they sit down. What is this?

A. While personal trainers cannot really determine for certain, a burning or cramping sensation in the calves felt soon after physical activity could be a sign of **intermittent claudication,** which may indicate peripheral artery disease (PAD). These are linked to heart disease. This condition results in a lack of blood flow to the legs due to the buildup of artery-clogging plaque. Sometimes the pain is felt in the thighs or buttocks also. Typically, the sensation starts after a few minutes of walking and stops soon after ceasing the activity. Because other factors may also cause this condition, people with this complaint should be referred to their physician, who can diagnose the problem.

Q. Are squats bad for the knees?

A. Several studies have found that squats are not innately harmful to the knees.[131] In fact, it is the official position of some fitness organizations that, if performed correctly, squats may even help reduce knee injuries by helping to stabilize the knee joint and to strengthen the muscles around that joint.[131] It is interesting to note that the original research on this dates back to the 1960s and was actually referring to deep squats, which go below 90°. It is also noteworthy that the deep-knee-squatting research has since been criticized by other investigators.[131] Nevertheless, more research is needed before this controversy is fully resolved.[185] For most clients, there is no need to squat below 90°.

Q. How much exercise do people need?

A. Generally, people should strive for between 30 and 60 minutes of moderate-intensity (e.g., 3–6 METs) aerobic exercise most day of the week.[1] For strength training, 2–3 days per week of exercise involving movements that target the major muscle groups is recommended. Thirty minutes is thought by some to be the minimum amount of exercise needed to maintain general health. Also, exercise does not all have to be done at the same time. For example, two 15-minute exercise sessions appears to be as good as a single 30-minute session. Some guidelines for losing weight call for up to 90 minutes of activity performed most days of the week.

Q. Do heavier people have slower metabolisms?

A. While possible, this is generally false. Heavier people and taller people tend to have higher resting metabolic rates than thinner and shorter people.

Q. Are natural vitamins better than synthetic vitamins?

A. Not necessarily. In some instances, synthetic vitamins are superior. Take folic acid, for example. Folic acid is the synthetic version of the B vitamin folate, and we absorb folic acid better than folate. For more insights on supplements, either see my website SupplementClarity.com or read my book, *Nutrition Essentials,* which is all about nutrition and sports nutrition and was written specifically for fitness professionals.

Q. What is the difference between a sprain and a strain?

A. A strain is an injury to a muscle or tendon (which connects muscles to bones), while a sprain is an injury to a ligament (which connects bones to each other). An easy way to remember the difference is to keep in mind that the word strain contains the letter "T" (for tendon). A sprain is a more acute injury, while a strain can be acute or may occur after repeated trauma (chronic). Both types of injuries are common in people who exercise. Acute versions of both may be helped with the "RICE" method (rest, ice, compression, elevation), but more severe types may require physical therapy or other medical interventions.

Q. Which is better: strength first or cardio first?

A. For most people—especially beginners—it does not matter since any form of physical activity is more beneficial than none at all. Some trainers look at this from the standpoint of which type of elevates post-exercise metabolic rate the most. One study noted that performing cardio before strength training resulted in a slightly greater metabolic rate (EPOC) than when strength training was performed first.[79] Another study hinted that performing cardio first might also elevate testosterone levels for a longer time than when the reverse order was performed.[190] This does not mean that doing cardio first is always best. For those who are beginners or those who have health problems, doing cardio first might be a safer bet. For those who have been working out for a while or are seeking weight loss, switching the order every couple of months will not hurt and may even have some benefits.

Q. Will weight lifting first make the body burn off its glycogen and help people burn fat better during cardio?

A. Weightlifting before cardio probably does not speed up the fat burning process if you are accustomed to that sequence of exercise. The primary fuel that the body uses during exercise is fat and carbohydrate. The average human body has enough energy in the form of glycogen (carbohydrate) to keep the person running for about 20 miles. People cannot burn off that much glycogen by lifting weights for 30–60 minutes. Since we need carbohydrates to burn fat, this is actually a good thing. Just as a fire needs oxygen to burn, fat needs carbohydrates to burn. Remember that "fat burning" does not necessarily equal "weight loss." As long as the calories consumed are fewer in number than the calories burned, it should not matter which form of exercise people do first in a workout.

Q. Does muscle weigh more than fat?

A. A pound of muscle and a pound of fat both weigh one pound. Muscle is denser than fat, and this is probably from the source of confusion. Because it is denser, muscle takes up less space.

Q. Can we turn fat into muscle?

A. No. They are two different types of tissues, and you cannot change one into the other.

Q. Can forced repetitions help weightlifters increase strength?

A. Forced repetitions occur when the lifter has help performing additional repetitions after he or she can no longer perform repetitions on his or her own. One study of basketball and volleyball players who trained for 6 weeks found that forced repetitions did not increase strength any more than when players lifted until muscular failure set in.[126] However, the limited amount of research on this topic makes drawing definitive conclusions about this practice difficult. Because forced repetitions carry a higher risk of injury, examine its usefulness within the context of a client's health, starting point, and goals before using.

Q. How does testosterone improve strength?

A. It appears that testosterone not only improves muscle protein synthesis, but at the same time slows protein breakdown. One study noted that heavy strength training improved muscle protein synthesis by 50% after 4 hours of exercise and by 109% 24 hours later![110] To naturally boost testosterone levels with resistance training, it is generally necessary to use heavier loads (e.g., 85% 1RM) coupled with short rest periods and moderate volumes (at least 4 sets). Obviously, this is an advanced protocol and not appropriate for beginners. People concerned about this should get their testosterone levels checked first to see if they are actually low.

Q. What are some natural ways to raise testosterone levels?

A. Both strength training and cardio will raise testosterone levels. Weight loss—even a few pounds—can raise levels too. With respect testosterone booster supplements, most contain unproven ingredients that lack evidence regarding their effectiveness. It is important to remind clients that advertisements for both prescription drugs and supplements try to make men feel they have "Low T." Before they spend their money, they should have their testosterone levels checked to see if it is, in fact, low. Normal testosterone levels range from about 300–1,000 ng/dL for men and 15–70 ng/dL for women.[194]

Q. Can muscles get stronger without growing larger?

A. Its possible. Remember that muscle hypertrophy and muscle strength do not always go hand-in-hand, and it is possible for muscles to grow stronger without a corresponding increase in muscle size. This appears to be especially true in prepubescent children, women, and in those who have worked out for at least two years.[109]

Q. Is weight-bearing exercise the same as weightlifting?

A. No. Weight-bearing activity occurs when you are supporting (bearing) your weight. Walking, for example, is a weight-bearing activity. Weight lifting, on the other hand, is moving an external resistance through a range of motion. Both can help strengthen bones, but since weight bearing usually involves the lower body, it tends to do little for the muscles and bones of the upper body.

Q. How much protein do we need?

A. Protein needs vary according many factors, including the age of the person and the source of protein. The RDA for healthy young people who do not exercise regularly is 0.8 grams per kilogram. That is 0.36 grams per pound. When it comes to exercise, research suggests that most people who exercise regularly should aim for between 1.2–1.8 g/kg/BW, which is about 0.6–0.9 grams per pound.[72, 182] Those who do primarily cardio should stay at the lower end, while those who primarily strength train may benefit from the higher end of this range. The often-repeated mantra, "1 gram per pound" for everybody has no basis in scientific fact. For more on sports nutrition, read my book *Nutrition Essentials*, available at my website, www.Joe-Cannon.com.

Q. When using creatine supplements, is the "loading phase" needed?

A. The loading phase typically consists of taking 20–25 grams of creatine per day for a week, followed by a maintenance phase of 2–5 grams per day. One interesting study noted that 1 month of using just 3 grams per day loaded muscles with as much creatine as did 1 week of using 20 grams per day.[80] Thus, according to this report, the loading phase may not be needed. The loading phase will quickly improve creatine storage and improve muscle power, but if you are not in a hurry, you probably do not need it.

Q. Do creatine supplements have any side effects?

A. The most consistently observed side effect is a gain in water weight. People tend to gain several pounds after a couple of weeks of using creatine supplements. Other side effects like kidney or liver damage and muscle or tendon tears have not been observed in well-designed clinical studies.

Q. Is creatine safe for kids?

A. Children are not miniature adults and may not respond the same as adults to creatine supplementation. Currently, there are no large-scale reliable studies of creatine supplements being used in humans under the age of legal consent. Thus, creatine supplements are not recommended for those under 18.

Q. Does creatine need to be cycled?

A. There is little evidence that people have to periodically cycle on and off creatine. I think that the main contributors to this idea are fears that that, over time, the body may "forget" to make creatine naturally if supplements continue to be taken. There is not much proof of this, though. That said, unless the person is performing activities that require power, creatine should not be needed. See the "Creatine" section of SupplementClarity.com for more information on this product.

Q. Is there any benefit to stretching between sets?

A. Yes. Stretching or performing light aerobic exercise between sets can enhance the clearance of metabolic acids and other metabolites from muscles, allowing them to recover more quickly. This can result faster recovery between sets.

Q. Does stretching make people weaker?

A. Several studies show that static stretching for 20–40 minutes before performing a bout of maximal exercise, like a 1RM squat, decreases muscle power. However, since most people do not stretch for this long prior to heavy weight lifting, this may not be a significant issue for most people who hire personal trainers. Also, static stretching for only 30 seconds does not appear to hinder athletic performance.[193]

Q. What is better for lowering blood pressure: high- or low-intensity exercise?

A. When it comes to lowering blood pressure, low-intensity exercise (RPE 2–3) tends to do a better job than high-intensity activity. The DASH Diet has also been shown to help blood pressure.

Q. How can a person have a low resting heart rate if they do not exercise regularly?

A. Usually, RHR decreases when people work out frequently. However, some medications like beta-blockers used to treat high blood pressure can also reduce it. In such instances, the use of the RPE scale and talk test are better than target heart rate for prescribing exercise intensity.

Q. Why can my client ride a bicycle for 60 miles but cannot run 1 mile?

A. While biking and running are both aerobic, biking works the muscles differently than running. For one thing, running is weight-bearing while biking is not. Remember the SAID principle: the body responds specifically to the exercise demands imposed on it. In other words, to be a better runner, do not bike—run.

Q. Are organic foods better?

A. Not necessarily. There are studies showing that organic foods have more of certain vitamins, while other studies show that they do not. When it comes to being healthy, most research supports the idea of eating more fruits and vegetables. The research does not differentiate between organic and non-organic foods. Thus, while eating organic foods will not hurt, whether or not they improve health more effectively is open to speculation. While organic foods are required to adhere to specific guidelines, be aware that some organic products in the frozen section of the supermarket may be high in fat and calories.

Q. Can vitamin C reduce muscle soreness?

A. There is very little evidence that vitamin C or other antioxidants reduce DOMS-related pain.[121] The best defense against DOMS is to progress slowly, starting with 1 set per exercise.

Q. To get stronger, do we have to feel sore after exercise?

A. Delayed muscle soreness (DOMS) does not have to be felt to improve muscle strength.[191] Also, reduced pain does not always mean that the muscle has fully recovered, either.

Q. Is exercise on an empty stomach best for weight loss?

A. The idea of working out in the morning before breakfast is that exercise will better target body fat and lead to more weight loss. The problem is that the research does not support this practice.[192] So far, most studies on this topic show that people burn more calories when they eat before exercise. Some research even suggests that exercise completed while in a fasted state increases protein breakdown, which in theory, may be detrimental to muscle growth.

Q. Where can I find more answers?

A. Go to www.Joe-Cannon.com and download my e-book, *The Personal Trainer's Big Book of Questions and Answers*. That book provides answers to well over 130 essential exercise, nutrition, and health questions that all trainers should know. My website also has a vast amount of other useful information as well.

Chapter 14

Special Populations

High Blood Pressure Guidelines

Key Points

➤ Also called hypertension. Defined as a consistent resting blood pressure of at least 140/90.

➤ Prehypertension is a BP of 120/80 (this used to be called "normal").

➤ High blood pressure is a major risk factor for stroke, the 4th leading cause of death.

➤ BP (especially systolic) tends to increase with age. All people should strive to maintain BP below 120/80.[164]

➤ Most cases have no known cause and are called idiopathic or primary hypertension. If the condition can be traced to another factor (obesity, etc.), it is called secondary hypertension.

➤ Not all cases can be controlled by diet and exercise alone.

➤ The following all increase risk: excess body weight, excess dietary sodium, reduced physical activity, and lack of fruits and vegetables in the diet.[164]

➤ Abbreviated as HTN by medical professionals.

General Guidelines for Hypertension[164]

➤ Lose weight if necessary. Strive for a BMI of 18.5/24.9.

➤ Stop smoking. Reduce saturated fat and cholesterol in the diet.

➤ Sodium intake should be no more than 1 teaspoon per day (2300 mg). For those over 51, it should be no more than 1500 mg per day.

➤ Increase potassium-rich foods (fruits and vegetables). Eat according to the DASH eating plan. DASH stands for "Dietary Approaches to Stop Hypertension" and is available online.

➤ Alcohol: Men should consume no more than 2 drinks per day. Women should drink no more than 1 drink per day.

➤ Exercise: Aim for at least 30 minutes of exercise most days of the week.

General Exercise Guidelines[141]

Type of Exercise	Exercise Guideline	Frequency, Intensity, Time
Aerobic	Large-muscle activities	RPE: 2–4 (0–10 scale) 30–60 min per day 3–7 days/wk Aim for burning 700–2000 calories per week
Strength Training	Circuit training	Low resistance, higher number of repetitions (e.g., 15–20 RM)

Comments & Suggestions

- If possible, take BP before and after exercise to gauge how exercise impacted BP.
- Do not exercise if BP is $\geq$ 200/115.
- Use RPE scale or Talk Test to gauge exercise intensity if the client is on medicines that slow heart rate.
- Weight training should not be the only type of exercise performed.
- Use overhead lifts with caution because of risks associated with the Valsalva maneuver.
- Avoid static contractions when possible.
- Avoid tight gripping of fitness equipment (e.g., treadmill handles and free weights).
- Avoid fast transfers from seated or supine positions to standing.
- Low-intensity exercise is better at lowering HTN than high-intensity exercise.
- For more information, visit the National Heart Lung and Blood Institute website at www.nhlbi.nih.gov.

High Cholesterol Guidelines

Key Points

- Hyperlipidemia refers to elevated levels of cholesterol and triglycerides.
- Hypercholesterolemia refers specifically to elevated levels of cholesterol (>200 mg/dL).
- Hypertriglyceridemia refers specifically to elevated levels of triglycerides (>150 mg/dL).
- HDL refers to high-density lipoprotein (good cholesterol); ≥40 mg/dL is appropriate.
- LDL refers to low-density lipoprotein (bad cholesterol); <100 mg/dL is appropriate.
- VLDL: Very low lipoprotein density. This is a type of LDL that has the most triglyceride. Normal levels range from 5–40 mg/dL.[175] As triglycerides lower, so does VLDL.[175]
- Elevated levels of LDL, cholesterol, and triglycerides are a risk factor for CAD.

General Exercise Guidelines

Type of Exercise	Exercise Guideline	Frequency, Intensity, time
Aerobic	Multi-joint activities	4–6 days per wk/40 min per session. RPE 2–4 (0–10 scale) or 11–16 (6–20 scale)
Strength Training	Circuit training	Light weights (e.g., 40–60% 1 RM), higher repetitions (e.g.,8–12 repetitions per set)

Comments & Suggestions

- Weight loss can often lower cholesterol and blood lipid levels.
- The optimal amount of exercise needed to impact lipids may vary from person to person. The main goal is to burn calories during exercise. Because cardio often burns more calories than strength training, it is often emphasized.
- An HDL of 60 mg/dL or more is a "negative risk factor" for heart disease, meaning that it lowers risk. Exercise—especially cardio—can increase HDL, but more HDL does not always mean less heart disease. LDL levels may be more important than HDL.
- If the person is using beta-blockers or other medications that lower RHR, RPE and/or the Talk Test are better than target heart rate for determining cardiovascular fitness.
- Determining 1RM may not be needed or advisable in this population because of other medical issues that the person may also have.
- For more information on cholesterol-lowering supplements, see my site, SupplementClarity.com.
- Adding a cardio station to the strength training circuit ramps up the aerobic component of the circuit.
- Besides exercise, it is important to limit dietary fat and cholesterol.
- For more information, visit the National Heart Lung and Blood Institute website at www.nhlbi.nih.gov.

Post-Heart-Attack Guidelines

Key Points

> ➢ Technically called myocardial infarction and abbreviated as "MI" by doctors.
> ➢ Coronary artery disease can lead to a heart attack and is often abbreviated as "CAD" by doctors.
> ➢ Heart attacks result when heart muscle dies from inadequate oxygen supply. This can result the buildup of artery-clogging plaque in blood vessels.

General Exercise Guidelines[141]

Type of Exercise	Exercise Guideline	Frequency, Intensity, time
Aerobic	Multi-joint movements	3–4 days per week RPE 2–6 (11–16 if using 6–20 scale), 20–40 min per session
Strength Training	Circuit training	2–3 days per week 1–3 sets of 10–15 repetitions

Comments & Suggestions

> ➢ People should be evaluated by a physician prior to starting an exercise program. Fitness trainers should obtain written permission from the physician with any special instructions prior to training.
> ➢ Doctors may quantify exercise capacity in terms of METs. Those with low fitness levels will probably be prescribed an exercise level of 5 METs or less.[141]
> ➢ Both warm-up and cool-down periods of about 10 minutes each are essential and may help stabilize heart rate before and after exercise.
> ➢ For resistance training, the loads lifted should be light to moderate (e.g., 10–15 repetitions per exercise).
> ➢ Some training recommendations call for starting a resistance training program at 50% 1RM, but this usually requires the determination of a person's 1RM, which may not be appropriate or safe.[177] Estimating 1RM from tables may likewise be inappropriate with this population.[177]
> ➢ Begin with only 1 set per exercise.
> ➢ When increasing weights, 2–5 pounds for upper body exercises and 5–10 pounds for lower body may be appropriate but can vary according to fitness level, age, and other health issues.[177]
> ➢ Rest periods between sets are generally 1.5–2 minutes but can vary according to fitness level.[177]
> ➢ Remind the person to breathe during resistance training. Avoiding the Valsalva maneuver in this way stabilizes BP.
> ➢ Rising too fast from seated, supine, or prone positions may result in a drop in BP (orthostatic hypotension) that can lead to fainting. Supervise when the person rises.
> ➢ People may have other issues to consider (e.g., diabetes or being overweight) when developing the exercise program.

➤ If the person is taking beta-blockers or other medications that slow HR, the RPE Scale is superior to heart rate when monitoring exercise intensity.[141]

➤ People who have had one heart attack may be at risk of another one. Be familiar with the signs of a heart attack and remember that high-intensity exercise increases this risk.

➤ People who complain of pain in their ankles or legs when walking, only to have it subside after ceasing activity, may have peripheral artery disease (abbreviated as PAD or PVD). Stationary bicycle or upper body aerobic exercise (e.g., UBE) may be an option for these individuals.

➤ For more information, visit the American Heart Association website at www.americanheart.org.

Diabetes Guidelines

Key Points

- Diabetes is defined as a metabolic disorder characterized by a failure to make the hormone insulin (type I) or the inability to use the insulin that is made (type II). Most cases are type II. Type I diabetics must inject insulin to survive. Both genetics and environmental factors play roles in the development of both types.
- Insulin is made in the beta cells of the pancreas and helps the body use sugar (glucose).
- Normal blood sugar is <100 mg/dL.
- Metabolic Syndrome is a cluster of conditions that increases risk for type II diabetes. Symptoms include abdominal obesity, reduced HDL, increased LDL and triglycerides, insulin resistance, and increased blood pressure. Exercise can improve metabolic syndrome.
- Hemoglobin A1c is a marker of average blood sugar levels over the last 3 months. A level of <6% is usually seen as normal.
- Type II diabetes appears to result from problems with insulin receptors. Lack of insulin receptors reduces the ability of insulin to work. Without insulin receptors, the body becomes "insulin resistant." That is, they make insulin but are resistant to its effects. Exercise makes insulin receptors work better.
- Type II diabetes may progress to type I if not treated. Type II diabetics may inject insulin as it becomes worse.
- Type I diabetes is caused by an autoimmune disorder. The immune system attacks the beta cells that make insulin. This decreases or shuts down insulin production.
- Diabetes may be accompanied by heart disease, vision problems, kidney problems, balance problems, and hypertension, to name a few.
- Hypoglycemia is low blood sugar. Signs can include rapid heart rate, sweating, anxiety, tremors, mental confusion, and ultimately loss of consciousness.
- Ketosis is an abnormal elevation in ketones. This results from burning the fat without the presence of carbohydrates (glucose). Ketosis upsets the acid/base balance of the body. If not treated, it can lead to death.

General Guidelines for Diabetes

- Lose weight if needed. Even modest weight loss can help, as can regular physical activity in general.
- Maintain appropriate blood sugar levels through proper nutrition, exercise, and drug therapy.

General Exercise Guidelines

Type of Exercise	Exercise Guideline	Frequency, Intensity, Time
Aerobic	Use large muscle groups	50–90% HR max 20–60 min per session Most days of the week.
Strength training	Interval training, including machines, free weights or a combination.	No official guidelines. Use caution with high intensity activity.
Flexibility	Improve balance and flexibility of joints.	No official guidelines.

Comments & Suggestions

- Do not exercise if blood sugar is >300 mg/dL.
- Client should be aware of the different types of insulin and when they are most effective at lowering blood sugar. They should avoid workouts when the insulin that they are using is most effective.
- Holding breath during strength training may damage already weakened blood vessels.
- If possible, measure blood sugar before and after exercise to gauge how exercise impacted blood sugar levels, especially when starting a new exercise program.
- Because balance and vision problems are common, stay with client at all times.
- Have carbohydrate snacks handy in case blood sugar dips too low.
- Remind clients that hypoglycemia may occur hours after the workout. Avoid exercising the area of the body that was injected with insulin.
- Diabetes can reduce testosterone levels and can cause erectile dysfunction.
- If diabetic passes out, it is safest to give the person sugar (carbohydrates). If hypoglycemia is the reason why the person passed out and insulin is administered, blood sugar will go even lower, which can be fatal. See my blog post, "Gym Emergency Procedures," available at Joe-Cannon.com, for more information.
- Increase exercise intensity gradually if athletic performance is a goal. Remember that higher intensities of exercise may increase blood sugar.
- Exercise alone may not be enough to help diabetes. Exercise usually has to be combined with weight loss in order to be beneficial.
- Loss of feeling in the feet (neuropathy) can lead to balance problems. Because of lack of feeling, injuries to the feet (blisters, broken bones, etc.) may not be noticed.
- See my blog post, "Natural Cure for Diabetes," available at Joe-Cannon.com, for more information.

Arthritis Guidelines

Key Points

- There are over 100 conditions classified as arthritis. The most common type is osteoarthritis. Another common type is rheumatoid arthritis.
- Osteoarthritis (OA or DJD) results from a wearing away of the joint cartilage. It can be caused by injury, ballistic sports participation, or obesity. Genetics may also play a role.
- Rheumatoid arthritis (RA) is thought to result from an autoimmune disorder in which immune cells attack the joints.
- Both OA and DJD result in deformity of the joints. The areas affected with arthritis will be weaker.

General Exercise Guidelines

Type of Exercise	Exercise Guideline	Frequency, Intensity, time
Aerobic	Mulit-joint movements	3–5 days per week RPE 2–6 5–30 min per day
Strength Training	Circuit training	2–3 days per week 2–12 repetitions Intensity varies with pain levels

Comments & Suggestions

- People often confuse osteoarthritis with osteoporosis.
- Because arthritis reduces mobility, people may have osteoporosis as well. Diabetes may also occur.
- Many will be deconditioned, requiring low levels of exercise at first. Thus, starting with light weights and very low repetitions may be warranted for strength training.
- Avoid high repetition, high-impact activities and those that use high levels of resistance.
- Activities that focus on balance, walking, and ADLs may help improve quality of life.
- Stretching is important to maintain pain-free ROM. However, overstretching joints may exacerbate pain. Never stretch to the point of pain. Static stretching is safest.
- Free weights can be used, but machines may be easier to work around limitations.
- Pool exercise can help improve CV endurance.
- When in doubt, increasing the amount of time for which the exercise is performed is safer than increasing the intensity of exercise.
- People with RA tend to have extended joint stiffness in the morning.[176] This may require extra warm-up time to compensate.
- Increased pain 1–2 hours after exercise may indicate that the person did too much.[176]
- It is probably safest to do cardio before strength training in a workout.
- For more information, visit the American Arthritis Foundation website at www.arthritis.org.

Fibromyalgia Syndrome Guidelines

Key Points

- A condition highlighted by widespread pain and stiffness felt throughout the body. Pain is felt at specific areas (tender points) of the body as well.
- Classified as a type of arthritis. The cause of fibromyalgia is unknown. Some research suggests that it may be related to a hypersensitivity of nerves that conduct feelings of pain in response to stimuli that normally are not painful.
- To be diagnosed, a person: 1.) Must be in pain for at least 3 months and 2.) Pain must be specific to at least 11 of 18 known tender points. All other causes must be ruled out as well.
- Tender points include those of the upper chest, the back of the head, the upper back, the neck, the elbows, the hips, and the knees. Fatigue and depression are also common in those suffering from fibromyalgia, as is numbness in the hands and/or feet.
- Pain varies according to emotions, stress, exercise, and lack of sleep.
- May be sensitive to cold, touch, and bright lights. Migraine headaches may also occur.
- Most sufferers are women, but men can also have fibromyalgia.
- People may not sleep well. Lack of quality sleep can increase feelings of pain and fatigue.

General Exercise Guidelines

Type of Exercise	Exercise Guideline	Frequency, Intensity, Time
Aerobic	Use large muscle groups	Low intensity—focus on time of exercise rather than intensity.
Strength training	Use light resistance	Light resistances—increase repetitions performed before increasing resistances used.
Flexibility	Stretch before exercise, during exercise, after exercise, and throughout the day	Stretch to mild discomfort only. Never stretch to pain.

Comments & Suggestions

- Focus on helping the person feel better and improve ADLs. Exercise programs should be gentle, especially at first.
- Pain levels can wax and wane, making periodized workouts difficult to create. Exercise intensity should not be the main focus of the program.
- Do not exercise to the point of muscle fatigue or failure, as this may make symptoms worse.
- Try not to cause DOMS, as this can make symptoms worse.
- Warm water pool exercise may help with pain levels.
- Some may have conditions other than fibromyalgia as well.
- Some may also have chronic fatigue syndrome, which is different than fibromyalgia, but symptoms can be very similar.
- For more information, visit the National Fibromyalgia Association website at www.fmaware.org.

Osteoporosis Guidelines

Key Points

> - Also known as brittle bone disorder.
> - Type I osteoporosis occurs between 50–70 yrs of age. Type II after 70 years of age.
> - Mostly affects postmenopausal women. Usually significant in men after age 70.
> - Poor or inadequate nutrition can promote osteoporosis at younger ages. By the age of 40, some bone loss has probably occurred. Building strong bones during youth reduces prevalence in old age.
> - Osteopenia is "pre-osteoporosis." Significant bone loss may have occurred but has not yet reached the point of osteoporosis. Osteopenia may progress to osteoporosis unless intervention occurs.
> - Common bones fractured from falls include the hips and wrist bones.
> - Osteoblasts are bone-making cells, osteocytes are mature bone cells, and osteoclasts are bone-eating cells.
> - Estrogen causes death to osteoclasts and extends the life of osteoblasts. After menopause, estrogen decreases and osteoclast activity ramps up, accelerating bone loss.
> - Risk factors include gender, ethnicity, genetics, age, thin bones, and lifestyle factors.
> - Life style factors include a lack of calcium and vitamin D, a lack of exercise, smoking, and excess consumption of alcohol.

General Exercise Guidelines[141]

Type of Exercise	Exercise Guideline	Frequency, Intensity, Time
Aerobic	Multi-joint activities	40–70% maximum heart rate 20–30 minutes per session, most days of the week
Strength training	Multi-joint activities. Machines or free weights appropriate.	2–3 sets of 50% 1RM or 70% 3RM, performed for 8 repetitions 2 days per week

Comments & Suggestions

> - If a novice has osteoporosis, start with lighter weights for the first few months to let the body adapt before loading it with heavier resistances. This will reduce injury.
> - Include balance and/or functional activities to improve hand-eye coordination and ADLs.
> - Some evidence suggests that crunches on the floor may increase prevalence of fractures to the spinal column.
> - For very deconditioned people, chair-based exercise programs may be needed.
> - Some people may have conditions other than osteoporosis. The guidelines for these other conditions may clash with guidelines for osteoporosis.
> - The characteristic curved upper back (hunch back) of many with osteoporosis may reduce the ability to breathe and thus impact exercise.

- Calcium supplements may be taken. Calcium carbonate is cheapest and has the most usable calcium per supplement. Calcium RDA is 1200–1500 mg/day. Have vitamin D levels checked before starting to take supplements.
- It may take at least a year before a noticeable impact on bone mass from exercise training is observed.
- For more information, visit the National Osteoporosis Foundation at www.nof.org.

Multiple Sclerosis Guidelines

Key Points

- Myelin is a fatty material that insulates and protects nerves and helps speed the transmission of nerve impulses in the central nervous system (CNS).
- MS results in an erosion (demyelination) of myelin. This causes a reduction in the speed of nerve transmission and a disruption of coordinated movements.
- The muscles of those with MS may contract involuntarily. This is referred to as **muscle spasticity.** This may result in awkward movements during walking and/or exercise. Treadmill exercise may be difficult for this population.
- As body temperature rises, muscle spasticity increases. Thus, frequent rest periods may be needed to maintain optimal body temperature.
- People with MS may also suffer from widespread pain.
- Symptoms can include disruptions to vision as well as problems with the bowels, coordination, fatigue, and pain.
- Symptoms can be relapsing in nature (coming and going). Most cases are of this type. Symptoms may also be progressive, in which case they may grow steadily worse over time.[178]
- Women are twice as likely to get MS as men.[178]
- MS is thought to result from an autoimmune disorder in which the immune system attacks the myelin covering. What causes the immune system to go awry is unknown. While a genetic link may exist, some research hints that exposure to environmental toxins (virus, bacteria, industrial toxin, etc.) early in life (before age 15) may predispose the person to MS later on.[179] Those living in high-risk areas who move to low risk areas before 15 are at lower risk of MS later in life.[179] Some also feel there may be a link between MS and low levels of vitamin D.[179]
- MS can occur at any age but mostly affects people between 15–50 years of age.[178]

General Exercise Guidelines

Type of Exercise	Exercise Guideline	Frequency, Intensity, time
Aerobic	Large muscle groups	3 days per week ≤ 70% HR max 30 min per session
Strength Training	Perform on different days than cardio	1–3 sets of 8–15 RM

Symptoms of Multiple Sclerosis*

Coordination	Muscle fatigue	Slurred speech
Attention span	Muscle atrophy	Urinary incontinence
Dizziness/ loss of balance	Muscle spasms	Uncontrolled rapid eye movements

*Partial list

Comments & Suggestions

- The goals of exercise are to slow the physical manifestations of MS and to maintain and/or improve fitness levels as well as help the person improve ADLs and quality of life.
- Exercising the hands and fingers and even making faces can be part of the exercise program.
- Depending on abilities, starting at a low level (e.g., 10 minutes) and gradually increasing time of exercise may be needed. Intermittent exercise may be needed in some people.
- Stretching, both passive and partner-assisted, can help improve circulation and may help muscle function.
- The environment should be free of any obstacles that can cause tripping. Likewise, wet floors may result in more falls.
- Some people with MS may not sweat very much, if at all. This can cause even moderate exercise to ramp up body temperature, which heightens muscle spasticity. If possible, keep room temperatures cool (66–70° F) and humidity as low as possible.
- While pool exercise may help, heated pools may exacerbate symptoms. Likewise, steam rooms and saunas should be avoided by those with MS.
- Some people with MS may be taking prednisone, an anti-inflammatory steroid that causes muscle weakness. It can also cause bone loss, fatigue, weight gain, and reduced wound healing. It can also cause extreme fluctuations in mood.[180]
- If balance and/or muscle spasticity are an issue, supervise closely during weight-bearing activity. Non-weight-bearing CV activity (e.g., the bike) may also help. Supervise when exiting fitness equipment.
- Wearing loose or light clothing can help keep the body cool and reduce muscle spasticity. Adequate hydration and weight loss may also help prevent body temperature elevations.
- Intense training may increase muscle spasticity.
- Symptoms may change daily, making exercise progressions difficult.
- Some may process information more slowly than usual. It may be necessary to repeat exercise instructions frequently. Positive reinforcement can help with frustration, depression, and exercise adherence.
- While free weights can be used, because of muscle spasticity and pain, machines may be safer. That said, other types of exercise equipment may be used if deemed appropriate.
- Avoid exercise to failure or exhaustion. Rest periods between sets of resistance training should be long enough to allow for recovery and to prevent core temperature elevations.
- Modify exercise programs according to MS flair ups and/or progression of the syndrome.
- Positive reinforcement should be used to foster exercise adherence.
- Remind the person to listen to his or her body and to be aware of possible signs of symptoms worsening with exercise.
- Reduce or stop exercise during flair-ups and resume the program when symptoms subside
- For more information, see the National Multiple Sclerosis Society website at www.nationalmssociety.org.

Prepubescent Children Guidelines

Key Points

➢ Discuss goals with parents—sports performance, sports injury reduction, weight loss, exercise instruction, etc.—before exercise training occurs.

➢ Exercise programs should include all aspects of fitness, including muscular and CV endurance, strength, and flexibility. Exercise programs should also be fun for the child.

➢ Adult exercise guidelines (e.g., 30–60 minutes of CV activity most days of the week) may not be appropriate for kids because of boredom and because aerobic adaptations to CV exercise may be less dramatic than in adults.[165] Games incorporating CV exercise may be better.

➢ Prepubescent boys and girls appear to increase strength to equal degrees.[5]

➢ Kids as young as 6 years of age have benefited from properly designed strength training programs.[166] There is no proof that a weight training program supervised by qualified instructors stunts the growth of kids. Damage to growth plates has not been reported.[5] However, if the program is not properly designed or supervised, injuries to growth plates may occur.

➢ The intensity of the program should not be too much for the child at his or her stage of development.

➢ Before puberty, most strength gains are due to neurological changes rather than increased muscle protein synthesis or hypertrophy.

General Exercise Guidelines

Type of Exercise	Exercise Guideline	Frequency, Intensity, time
Aerobic	No official guidelines. Multi-joint activities (games, treadmill, walking, jogging) are suggested.	No official guidelines. Interval training may mimic how kids play in the real world.
Strength training	Multi-joint and single-joint activities. Machines, free weights, body weight exercises.	Light resistance (12–20 repetitions) 2–3 days per week

Comments & Suggestions

➢ Consider the maturity level when developing an exercise program. Can the child follow directions?

➢ Be someone whom the child feels comfortable approaching. Be open to the child's concerns and possible fears about exercise. Always include a 5–10 minute warm-up prior to exercise.

➢ It is usually not necessary to determine RM values. Focus on exercise technique and form rather than weight lifted. Resistances lifted for 12–20 repetitions are usually adequate.

➢ Exercise should be fun, especially for young kids. Games may be preferable for some.

➢ Evidence suggests that properly designed resistance training programs can improve bone density, aerobic fitness, lower cholesterol levels, improve skill performance, and improve body composistion.[5]

➢ Kids take longer to sweat and tend to sweat less than adults. As such, kids may be at greater risk of hyperthermia. Overweight kids may be especially prone because of the insulating effect of excess body weight. Remember to take time to hydrate.

➢ Educate the child that the maximum amount of weight lifted is not important. Focus on long-term health benefits. Speaking in language that the child can understand and using ideas and phrases common to younger generations may enhance the child's exercise education and long-term adherence to exercise.

➢ If necessary, discuss with parents the notion that supplements are not needed and usually lack proof that they actually work.

Frail and Older Adult Guidelines

Key Points

- "Frail" is defined as lacking the strength or endurance to perform 2 or more ADLs. Someone who has sarcopenia may also be classified as "frail."
- It is possible to be young and frail, just as it is possible to be older and not frail.
- Anything that limits mobility can lead to being frail.
- Frailty may also result in other issues (diabetes, obesity, etc.).
- Americans are growing older. Most people in nursing homes are also over 85. Fewer than 1% of those over age 85 do resistance training.
- Proper exercise can help slow and may sometimes reverse many aspects of the aging process.

General Exercise Guidelines

Type of Exercise	Exercise Guideline	Frequency, Intensity, time
Aerobic	Low intensity. Progress as tolerated.	5–60 min/day 3–5 days/week Low intensity
Strength training	Start with low intensity. Progress as strength improves.	20 min per session 3 days per week Intensity level varies among people

Comments & Suggestions

- There is no universal exercise guideline that can be applied to all people who are frail or elderly. The trick is to look at the whole person—likes, dislikes, abilities, health history, ADLs, limitations, and goals—and find something that works for him or her.
- Balance may be an issue and something to incorporate into the exercise program.
- Reducing the risk of falling through exercise and proper movement mechanics can help improve the quality and quantity of life.
- With older individuals, longer rest periods (e.g., 2–5 min) may be needed between sets.
- For older individuals or those using medications that lower HR, the Talk Test and/or RPE Scale are preferable to HR when estimating exercise intensity.
- Do not worry about target heart rate in older individuals.
- For those with blood pressure issues, avoid static and isometric exercises.
- Avoid ballistic movements, as they may increase injury.
- Functional training may, in some instances, help improve ADLs.
- Because of sarcopenia, frail people will move more slowly and take longer to react due to reductions in type II fiber density. If possible, targeting type II fibers may improve life quality.
- Frail or older individuals may not consume adequate or quality calories or enough fluids.
- Older adults may have a reduced sensation of thirst, which may lead to dehydration, overheating, and reduced exercise capacity. They may also eat fewer calories and less protein and may be less efficient at producing muscle protein, a process called **anabolic resistance.**

- Healthy older adults with no medical issues can lift heavy weights.[77] Varying the resistance seems to improve strength more than constantly lifting heavy weights.[77]
- Because of weakened condition, exercising to exhaustion is not recommended.

Pregnancy Guidelines

Key Points

- Moderate exercise is safe for women with uncomplicated pregnancies.[167] One of the main goals of the exercise program is to prepare women for the demands of labor and childbirth.
- Sedentary women who start an exercise program while pregnant must obtain physician's permission first.[1] Progress slowly and within the client's comfort level.[167]
- Women who exercise during pregnancy experience less low back pain compared to sedentary women.[168]
- Fetal size does not appear to be affected by moderate exercise training during pregnancy.[167] Intense exercise (1–2.5 hours/day) may result in lower fat mass of babies.[169]
- Gestational diabetes may occur as a result of increased blood sugar during pregnancy.

Absolute Contraindications to Exercise While Pregnant[167, 174]

Pregnant with 3 or more babies	Pregnancy-induced high blood pressure
Preeclampsia/eclampsia	Bleeding in the 2nd or 3rd trimesters
Weak cervix	Women at risk of premature labor
Smoking /alcohol abuse	Previous spontaneous abortion

Possible Contraindications to Exercise That Require Physician's Approval[167, 174]

Any cardiovascular problems	Mother is underweight or has eating disorder
Low fitness level	Anemia
Type I or II diabetes	Any significant medical issues

General Exercise Guidelines[167, 174]

Type of Exercise	Exercise Guideline	Frequency, Intensity, time
Aerobic	Low intensity	If sedentary, start with 15 min, 3 days/week. Progress to 30 min, 4 days/week. Work until point of fatigue, never exhaustion.
Strength Training	Train for muscular endurance	Light weight. Increase repetitions/sets as tolerated.

Comments & Suggestions

➤ Goals for exercise should be to train for muscular endurance, focusing on the muscles involved in labor. Goals may include maintaining ADLs, improving posture during pregnancy, reducing low back pain, and strengthening weight bearing muscles.[173]

➤ Do not exercise to failure or exhaustion. Cease exercise when fatigued.[1]

➤ Machines may, in some instances, be safer than free weights. Pregnancy may preclude the use of some machines because of increased abdominal girth and/or restricted ROM.

➤ Avoid crunches after the first trimester. Crunches may cause diastasis, or tearing of the rectus abdominis muscle.

➤ After the first trimester, avoid exercises that place the woman in the supine (lying on the back) position, as this can reduce blood pressure and cardiac output and block blood flow to the baby.

➤ Water-based exercise is usually appropriate for this population and helps reduce maternal core temperature and edema and facilitates blood flow to the baby. Scuba diving, however, should be avoided throughout the pregnancy.

➤ Sedentary women who start an exercise program while pregnant may be at greater risk of medical issues than those who are regular exercisers.

➤ Avoid ballistic-type exercises and those that require excessive balance with added resistances (e.g., lunges, squats, stiff-leg dead lifts).

➤ Avoid activities that require long periods of motionless standing.

➤ Balance issues may arise because of distended abdominal girth. Avoid activities that require fast changes in direction.

➤ Because of hormonal fluctuations, joints may become hyper flexible (laxity), resulting in increased risk of injury.

➤ As pregnancy progresses, exercise may become noticeably more difficult. Adjust exercise intensity accordingly.

➤ Excessive low back inward curvature (lordosis) may result in back pain. Excessive curvature of the upper back (kyphosis) may cause a rounding of the shoulders.

➤ RHR may rise by 10–15 bpm when pregnant.

➤ Both the Talk Test and RPE Scale can be used to monitor exercise exertion during pregnancy.[167]

➤ Total blood volume may increase in pregnant women by as much as 40% above normal. This could lead to swelling in the arms or legs, nose and gum bleeding, varicose veins, and headaches.

➤ At least 300 extra calories per day may be needed during pregnancy because of increased metabolic rate. Women who exercise may need extra calories.[167]

➤ Exercise in hot and/or humid environments is not recommended, as it may elevate body temperature. This effect may be more pronounced in untrained women.[170]

➤ Maintain adequate hydration, as this can help maintain proper core temperature.

➤ Pain in the groin or anterior thigh could, in theory, indicate osteoporosis of the hip.[171] Consult a physician for diagnosis.

➤ Fitness testing is not necessary for pregnant women.[174]

➤ Physician approval to exercise may be withdrawn if medical issues arise during pregnancy.

➤ After delivery, exercise should be resumed gradually. At least 6 weeks may be needed before the woman's body returns to the pre-pregnancy state.[1]

Reasons for Stopping Exercise and Seeking Immediate Medical Attention[1]

Fluid discharge from vagina	Unknown loss of consciousness or fainting	Chest pain, rapid HR, fatigue, or unknown abdominal pain
Bloody discharge from vagina	Persistent increase in BP or HR after exercise stops	Uterine contractions
Severe headache, vision disruption	Swelling/pain/redness in one calf	Abrupt swelling of ankles, face, or hands

Visual Impairments Guidelines

Key Points

➢ Deficits in vision can be caused by a number of factors ranging from cataracts to glaucoma, age-related macular degeneration (AMD), and head trauma, to name a few.

General Exercise Guidelines

Type of Exercise	Exercise Guideline	Frequency, Intensity, time
Aerobic	No official guidelines. Large muscle groups.	20–60 minutes, most days of the week
Strength Training	No official guidelines	2–3 days per week. Intensity and time vary as tolerated according to fitness level

Comments & Suggestions

➢ If visual impairment is the only health issue to consider, these people are considered apparently healthy and can be trained similarly to healthy, sighted individuals with few restrictions. If other issues exist, work within established guidelines for those conditions.

➢ Those with vision issues will likely also have balance detriments. The trainer should stay with the individual and, if needed, physically guide him or her through the workout.

➢ People with vision impairments may have low CV endurance and strength due to reduced ability to exercise alone. This may lead to various associated conditions such as weight gain and type II diabetes. Heart disease is possible as well.

➢ Individuals may suffer from a fear or anxiety of unfamiliar surroundings such as the gym. Trainers should be aware of this and work to foster a bond of trust with the person.

➢ Verbal and physical cues or instructions are especially important if using free weights. The trainer should help the lifter with the lift-off and re-racking of the weight.

➢ If blindness was caused by physical trauma (detached retina) or if the person recently had cataract surgery, avoid activities that are high-impact.[141] Likewise, heavy weightlifting and intense cardio are not advised after recent eye surgery. Facial deformity may also be present following physical trauma, which may further foster feelings of anxiety on the part of the individual.

➢ If exercising in a health club, the trainer should walk the person around the facility to make them aware of landmarks, emergency exits, stairs, locker rooms, and other important features before training begins.

➢ If working out alone in a pool, the facility should place an audible sound (e.g., radio) at the shallow end of the pool to help the person differentiate the deep from the shallow end.

➢ Exercise should stop and the person referred to an eye doctor if any worsening of vision occurs during exercise.

➢ Remember that visual issues can be caused by diabetes. In such instances, train according to the guidelines for that condition.

Glossary

Abduction. To move a body part away from the body. Sometimes called AB-duction.

Actin. A muscle protein. One of the myofilaments found in myofibrils.

Acute. In exercise, usually refers to a short-term change. *Chronic* refers to long-term change.

Adduction. To move a body part closer to the body. Sometimes called AD-duction.

ADL. Activity of daily living. Tasks performed on a regular basis. Walking and going to the bathroom are ADLs. IADLs are instrumental activities of daily living. IADLs refer to paying bills, cooking, laundry, and shopping.

Aerobic Exercise. Exercise that uses oxygen to generate energy (ATP). Also called cardiovascular exercise.

Anabolic Resistance. Reduced protein synthesis that occurs with aging. Also see *sarcopenia*.

Anaerobic Exercise. Exercise that does not require oxygen to make energy (ATP).

Antagonist Muscle. The muscle or muscles that oppose the prime mover. Antagonists help slow down joint movement and overall help reduce joint injury. See also *prime mover*.

Apparently Healthy. A term used to describe people with no apparent health issues.

Articular Cartilage. Joint cartilage found at the ends of bones.

ATP. Adenosine Triphosphate. The body's ultimate energy molecule.

BPM. Abbreviation for "beats per minute."

BMD. Bone mineral density. Osteoporosis results in a reduction in BMD.

BMI. Body mass index.

BMR. Basal Metabolic Rate. The lowest metabolism possible. See also *RMR*.

Body Composition. The amount of fat and fat-free mass that a body contains.

Borg Scale. Also called "RPE scale." A 0–10 scale used to estimate exercise intensity.

Carbohydrate. Carbohydrates are sugars. The main energy source used during exercise.

Cardiovascular Exercise. Aerobic exercise.

Closed Grip. In weight lifting, a closed grip occurs when the thumbs are wrapped around the bar of the free weight or handle of the weight machine.

Concentric Muscle Action. In weightlifting, the phase of a muscle contraction where the weight is lifted. Also called "positives." See also *eccentric*.

Core. In exercise, all of the muscles of the trunk.

CNS. Central nervous system. Consists of the brain and spinal cord.

COPD. Chronic Obstructive Pulmonary Disorder. Lung disease that makes it hard to breathe, like emphysema or chronic bronchitis. COPD is the fourth-leading cause of death. Smoking is the primary risk factor for COPD.

CPT. Certified Personal Trainer.

Creatine Phosphate. An energy source that helps regenerate ATP during periods of intense physical activity.

CRP. C-Reactive Protein. Elevations of CRP may be linked to heart disease.

DOMS. Delayed Onset Muscle Soreness.

Diastolic Blood Pressure. The pressure of the blood on the walls of the blood vessels when the heart is in its filling phase. See also *systolic BP* and *blood pressure.*

Eccentric Muscle Action. In weightlifting, the phase of a muscle contraction where the weight is lowered. Also called "negatives." See also *concentric.*

Ejection Fraction. The percentage of blood pumped from the heart with each heartbeat.

Electrolytes. Elements that allow electrical impulses to be transmitted in biological systems. Sodium, potassium, calcium, and chloride are examples of electrolytes.

EPOC. Excessive Post-exercise Oxygen Consumption. EPOC refers to the elevation in metabolism that occurs after exercise. The older name is "oxygen debt." See also *NEAT.*

Fast-Twitch Muscle. Type II muscle fibers.

FITT Principle. Frequency, Intensity, Time, and Type of exercise.

Free Weight. Barbells and dumbbells.

Glucogenolysis. The breakdown of glycogen to glucose.

Gluconeogenesis. The making of sugar (glucose) from non-carbohydrate substances (e.g. protein).

Glucose. Blood sugar. Normal blood sugar is less than 100 mg/dL.

Glycogen. Storage form of glucose

Glycogenesis. The making of glycogen.

Glycolysis. The chemical pathway responsible for the breakdown of sugar (glucose) for energy (ATP) that does not require oxygen. Glycolysis is an anaerobic energy system.

Gram. Unit of weight in the metric system. There are 28 grams in 1 ounce.

HDL. High-density lipoprotein. The so-called "good" cholesterol. See also *LDL* and *cholesterol.*

Hemoglobin A1c. A marker of long-term blood sugar levels (~3 months). Elevated levels increase risk of heart disease. Also abbreviated as "HbA1c."

Homeostasis. Refers to maintaining an internal balance. Our ability to survive as our environment changes is ultimately due to our body's ability to keep the status quo.

HR. Heart Rate. Maximum heart rate is abbreviated as "Max HR" or "HR max."

Hyperplasia. Refers to an increase in cell number.

Hypertension. High blood pressure. Abbreviated as "HTN."

Hypertrophy. An increase in size.

Hypoglycemia. Low blood sugar levels.

Idiopathic. A condition that has no known cause.

Isometric Muscle Action. A type of muscle action in which the muscle does not change in length while force is applied to it. Also called "static contractions."

Isotonic Muscle Action. A type of muscle action where the tension on the muscle remains constant while the muscle changes its length. Composed of two phases called "concentric" and "eccentric."

Kilogram. One kilogram = 1,000 grams. One kilogram (1 kg) is equal to about 2.2 pounds.

Krebs Cycle. The chemical reaction series that involves the aerobic breakdown of fat.

Lactate. A metabolic byproduct of glycolysis made during the anaerobic breaking down sugar (glucose) for energy (ATP). Production coincides with the burning sensation during felt during intense exercise. Sometimes called "lactic acid," but they are not the same thing.

LDL. Low-density lipoprotein. Also called "bad" cholesterol.

Macronutrient. Nutrients that make up the greatest amount of our diet. Proteins, fats, and carbohydrates are the macronutrients.

MET. Metabolic equivalents. 1 MET is equal to 3.5 milliliters of oxygen per kilogram of body weight per minute. METs are another way to measure exercise intensity.

Metabolic Syndrome. Several symptoms that tend to occur together and that appear to increase risk of type II diabetes. Used to be called "syndrome X."

Metabolism. The total of all the chemical reactions (anabolic + catabolic) in the body. Also, the speed at which we burn calories.

M.I. Abbreviation for "myocardial infarction." A heart attack.

Mitochondria. A region of the cell where fat is broken down to generate energy (ATP).

Multi-joint Exercise. A movement that uses many muscles simultaneously. Also called a "compound exercise." An example is the leg press. See also *single joint exercise*.

Myofibril. Basically, complexes of myosin and actin proteins (and other proteins) that make up muscle fibers.

Myoglobin. An oxygen-carrying compound in muscle cells that is similar to hemoglobin.

Myosin. A muscle protein. One of the myofilaments found in myofibrils.

NEAT. Non-exercise activity thermogenesis. Any activity other than exercise that burns calories. Examples include shopping, gardening, and working. See also *EPOC*.

Neutral Grip. In weight lifting, when the hands are facing each other.

Obese. Excessively overweight. A BMI greater than 30 is considered obese.

Osteoporosis. A disease in which bones become brittle and break easily. Osteoporosis affects both men and women.

OT. Occupational Therapist. See also *PT*.

Overtraining Syndrome. A phenomenon that occurs when people regularly exercise to exhaustion and do not get enough rest between exercise sessions.

Oxygen Consumption. The amount of oxygen that can be used to make energy aerobically. Higher consumptions are associated with greater aerobic fitness.

Periodization. An exercise protocol in which an exercise program is divided into different cycles or phases. Different goals are addressed in each of the various periodization phases. The main objectives of periodization are to maximize training goals while reducing injury.

pH. A 0–14 acidity scale. Lower numbers mean more acidity. Higher numbers mean more alkalinity.

Power. Power is explosive strength. Power does not last long (e.g. 20–30 seconds). Strength and power are not the same. Strength generally lasts for 2–5 minutes.

Preeclampsia. High blood pressure occurring during pregnancy and post-pregnancy. Eclampsia refers to seizures during pregnancy.

Prehypertension. A consistent resting blood pressure that is 120/80 mm Hg–139/89 mm Hg.

Prime Mover. The muscle primary responsible for the movement. Also called the "agonist."

Prone. Anatomical position where the person is laying on his or her stomach. The pronated position is also when the palms of the hands are facing downward. See also *supine*.

Protein. One of the macronutrients. Proteins are made of smaller units called amino acids.

PT. Physical Therapist. See also *OT*.

RD. Registered Dietitian.

Repetition. One complete cycle of an exercise. For example, lifting a weight 12 times means that you performed 12 repetitions. Abbreviated as "rep." See also *set*.

Rhabdomyolysis. Muscle fiber death. Can be caused by too much exercise.

RHR. Resting heart rate.

RM. Repetition Maximum. The most weight that one can lift for a certain number of times with good lifting technique.

RMR. Resting Metabolic Rate.

ROM. Range of motion.

RPE Scale. Ratings of Perceived Exertion Scale. Also known as the Borg Scale.

Sarcomere. The basic unit of muscle contraction.

Sarcopenia. Loss of muscle as we grow older.

Sedentary. One who does not exercise regularly.

Selectorized Machine. Type of strength training machine in which the resistance can be selected (e.g. inserting a pin into a weight stack).

Set. A group of repetitions.

Single-Joint Exercise. An exercise that uses smaller amounts of muscles.

Skeletal muscle. Muscles that are attached to the skeleton. The biceps, for example, are skeletal muscles.

Slow-Twitch Muscle. Type I muscle fibers.

Soft Lock-Out. A soft lock-out occurs when the joint is nearly straight but not totally locked out.

Special Populations. Phrase used for anyone who has a special need. Examples include those with osteoporosis, high blood pressure, or heart disease.

Spotting. A spotter is a lifting partner (or trainer) who spots and corrects errors in exercise technique and/or assists the lifter performing the movement.

Sticking Point. The most difficult part of a weight lifting movement.

Supine. Anatomical position in which one is lying on the back. Supination also occurs when the palms of the hands are facing upward. See also *prone*.

Synergist Muscle. A helper muscle. A synergist muscle acts in synergy or cooperation with the prime mover to accomplish the task at hand. See also *prime mover*.

Systolic Blood Pressure. The pressure of the blood on the walls of the blood vessels when the heart is in its contraction phase.

Thermic Effect of Food. The amount of calories we use digesting food.

THR. Target Heart Rate.

Triglyceride. Another name for fat. Triglycerides are stored in fat cells and released into the blood when needed, such as during exercise.

Type I Muscle Fibers. Slow-twitch fibers.

Type II Muscle Fibers. Fast-twitch fibers.

Valsalva Maneuver. Holding the breath during exercise.

VO$_2$. The volume of oxygen used to make energy aerobically. Used as a measure of exercise intensity and aerobic fitness. See also *oxygen consumption* and *METs*.

Volume. In exercise, defined as the weight x repetitions x sets. Example, performing 2 sets of an exercise at 100 pounds for 10 repetitions is 100 x 10 x 2 = 2,000 pounds.

Sample Health History Form

Today's Date _____
Name _____
Address _____
City / State / Zip _____
Phone (H) _____
Phone (W) _____
Primary Email _____
Date of Birth _____
Age _____
Weight (lb.) _____   Height (in) _____

Emergency Contact Information

Name _____   Relationship _____
Phone (H)_____   Phone (W) _____

Name of Personal Physician

Dr. Name _____
Office address _____
Office Telephone _____

Personal Health History

Do you now have or have you had in the past, any of the following conditions or syndromes?

1. Heart attack	yes	no
2. Chest pain at rest	yes	no
3. Chest pain during physical activity	yes	no
4. Heart surgery	yes	no
5. Irregular heartbeat	yes	no
6. Do you have a pacemaker	yes	no
7. Other heart problems not listed above	yes	no

8. If yes, please explain _____
_____

9. High cholesterol	yes	no
10. High triglycerides	yes	no
11. Stroke	yes	no
12. Diabetes	yes	no
13. If yes, what type do you have:	Type I	Type II
14. Osteoarthritis	yes	no

15. Rheumatoid arthritis	yes	no
16. Asthma	yes	no
17. Emphysema	yes	no
18. Currently pregnant	yes	no
19. Cancer	yes	no
20. Recent surgery	yes	no
21. History of neck problems	yes	no
22. History of back problems	yes	no
23. History of knee problems	yes	no
24. History of shoulder problems	yes	no
25. Hearing problems	yes	no
26. Vision problems	yes	no
27. Problems maintaining balance	yes	no
28. Osteoporosis	yes	no
29. High blood pressure	yes	no
30. Other medical problems not listed above	yes	no

31. If yes, please explain _____
32. When was your last physical? _____
33. Do you currently smoke?   yes   no
34. Do you ever experience spells of severe dizziness?   yes   no
35. Have you undergone physical therapy in the last 2 years? _____
36. Do you ever experience shortness of breath? _____
37. Do you have any other health issue not mentioned above? _____

Family Medical History

Do you have a family history of any of the following?

Diabetes	yes	no
Cancer	yes	no
Osteoporosis	yes	no
Heart disease	yes	no
Stroke	yes	no
Obesity	yes	no

Are both parents still alive?   yes   no

If not, how old were they and what was the cause of death? _____

Medications

To the best of your knowledge, please list all medications you are taking and the reasons you are taking them _____
_____
_____

References

1. ACSM's Guidelines for Exercise Testing and Prescription, 6th edition. Lippincott Williams & Williams.

2. Heyward, VH (1991). Advanced Fitness Assessment & Exercise Prescription. Second edition. Human Kinetics.

3. Heyward, VH (1997). Advanced Fitness Assessment & Exercise Prescription. Third edition. Human Kinetics.

4. Golding LA, Myers CA and Sinning WE (1989). Y's Way to Physical Fitness, 3rd edt. Human Kinetics.

5. Earl RW & Baechle TR (2004). NSCA's Essentials of Personal Training. Human Kinetics.

6. No authors. One Rep Maximum. wikipedia.org/wiki/One_rep_maximum (accessed 11/26/06).

7. No authors. Department of Health and Human Services. www.surgeongeneral.gov/topics/obesity/calltoaction/fact_consequences.htm (accessed 12/5/06).

8. McArdle, W. D., Katch, F. I., Katch, V. L. (1999). Sport & Exercise Nutrition. Lippincott, Williams & Wilkins.

9. Broeder CE (1997). Assessing body composition before and after resistance or endurance training. Medicine and Science in Sports and Exercise, 29,5, 705-712.

10. Maddalozzo, G. F..et al. (2002). Concurrent validity of the BOD POD and dual nergy x-ray absorptiometry techniques for assessing body composition in young women. Journal of the American Dietetic Association, 102,11,1677 1679.

11. Utter, A.C. et al. (2003). Evaluation of air displacement for assessing body composition of collegiate wrestlers. Medicine and Science in Sports and Exercise, 35,3, 00-505.

12. Vescovi, J. D. et al. (2002). Evaluation of the BOD POD for estimating percent fat in female college athletes. Journal of Strength and Conditioning Research, 16, 4, 599-605.

13. Vescovi, J.D. et al. (2001). Evaluation of the BOD POD for estimating percentage body fat in a heterogeneous group of adult humans. European Journal of Applied Physiology, 85, 3-4, 326-332.

14. Lockner D.W. et al. (2000). Comparison of air-displacement plethysmography, hydrodensitometry, and dual X-ray absorptiometry for assessing body composition of children 10 to 18 years of age. Annals of the New York Academy of Science, 904, 72-78.

15. Jouven X et al (2005).Heart rate profile during exercise as a predictor of sudden death. New England Journal of Medicine, 12,352 (19), 1951-1958.

16. Brooks D (1997). Program Design for Personal Trainers. Moves International.

17. Chobanian AV et al (2003). The seventh report of the joint national committee on prevention, detection, evaluation and treatment of high blood pressure. The JNC 7 report. JAMA, 289,19,2560-2572.

18. No author. Heart. How It Works. American Heart Association. www.americanheart.org/presenter.jhtmL?identifier=4642 (accessed 1/8/07)

19. MacReady, N. Drugs and Athletes: It's All About the Gold. www.webmd.com/content/article/36/1728_61278.htm (accessed 1/12/07)

20. CDC.gov. Prevention Information and Advice for Athletes. www.cdc.gov/mrsa/community/team-hc-providers/advice-for-athletes.htmL (accessed 7/20/14)

21. Rhoades RA, Tanner GA (editors) (2003). *Medical Physiology*, 2nd ed., Lippincott Williams & Wilkins.

22. Stryer, L (1988). Biochemistry, 3rd edt W.H. Freeman and Company.

23. No author. An Introduction to Carbon Monoxide. Environmental Protection Agency. www.epa.gov/iaq/co.htmL#Health%20Effects%20Associated%20with%20Carbon%20Monoxide (accessed 1/16/07).

24. Guyton AC et al. (1996). Textbook of Medical Physiology, 9th edition.

25. Howley ET and Franks BD (1997). Health Fitness Instructor's Handbook. 3rd edition. Human Kinetics.

26. Persinger R et al (2004). Consistency of the talk test for exercise prescription. Medicine and Science in Sports and Exercise, 36,9, 1632-1636.

27. Rubal BJ et al (1987). Effects of physical conditioning on the heart size and wall thickness of college women. Medicine and Science in Sports and Exercise 19,5,423-429

28. Kiens B et al (1993). Skeletal muscle substrate utilization during submaximal exercise in man.: Effects of endurance training. Journal of Physiology, 469,459-478.

29. Powers SK and Howley ET (1990). Exercise Physiology: Theory and Application to Fitness and Performance. Second edition. Brown & Benchmark.

30. Fox E, Bowers R and Foss M (1993). The Physiological Basis for Exercise and Sport. Fifth edition. Brown & Benchmark.

31. Sugiura H et al (2002). Effects of long term moderate exercise and increase in number of daily steps on serum lipids in women. Randomized control trial. BMC Women's Health, 2:3 www.biomedcentral.com/1472-6874/2/3 (accessed 2/13/07).

32. Pate, RR., et al (1995). Physical activity and public health: A recommendation from the Centers for Disease Control and Prevention and the American College of Sports Medicine. *JAMA*. 273:402–407. 1995.

33. Quinn TJ et al. (2006). Two short daily activity bouts vs. one long bout: are health and fitness improvements similar over twelve and twenty-four weeks? Journal of Strength and Conditioning Research, 20,1, 130-135.

34. Adams AK et al. (2002). The role of antioxidants in exercise and disease prevention. Physician and Sports Medicine, 30,5 www.physsportsmed.com/issues/2002/05_02/adams.htm (accessed 2/13/07).

35. No authors. General physical activities defined by level of intensity. Center for Disease Control and Prevention. www.cdc.gov/nccdphp/dnpa/physical/pdf/PA_Intensity_table_2_1.pdf (accessed 2/14/07).

36. Ainsworth BE. (2002, January) The Compendium of Physical Activities Tracking Guide. Prevention Research Center, Norman J. Arnold School of Public Health, University of South Carolina. http://prevention.sph.sc.edu/tools/compendium.htm (accessed 2/14/07).

37. Maxwell AJ et al. (2002). Randomized trial of a medical food for the dietary management of chronic, stable angina. Jouirnal of the American College of Cardiology, 39, 37-45.

38. Cannon, J (2006). Nutritional Supplements: What Works and Why. A Review from A to Zinc and Beyond. Available at Joe-Cannon.com.

39. Nieman, DC (1998). The Exercise-Health Connection. Human Kinetics.

40. US Bureau of Labor and Statistics. www.ubs.gov (accessed July 18 2014).

41. Cerny FT and Burton HW (2001). Exercise Physiology for Health Car Professionals. Human Kinetics.

42. Wilmore JH & Costill DL ((1994). Physiology of Sport and Exercise. Human Kinetics.

43. Physical Activity and Health. Chapter 3: Physiologic Responses and Long-Term Adaptations to Exercise. Center for Disease Control and Prevention. www.cdc.gov/nccdphp/sgr/chap3.htm (accessed 2/22/07).

44. Peters, R.K., Bateman, E.D. (1983). Ultramarathon running an upper respiratory track infections. South_African Medical Journal, 64, 582-584.

45. Kohut M, et al. (2002). Exercise and psychosocial factors modulate immunity to influenza vaccine in elderly individuals. Journal of Gerontology, 57A(9): M557–M562.

46. Fiscella, C. (2005). The Lumbar Spine. IDEA Fitness Journal. May, 34-37.

47. No authors. Your high blood pressure questions answered – blood pressure and exercise. American Heart Association www.americanheart.org/presenter.jhtmL?identifier=3034814 (accessed 3/8/07).

48. Newham, et al. (1987). Repeated high - Force Eccentric Exercise: Effects on Muscle Pain and Damage. Journal of Applied Physiology 63,41381-1386.

49. Margetic S et al (2002). Leptin: a review of its peripheral actions and interactions. International Journal of Obesity 26 1407–1433.

50. Kojima, M. et. al. (1999). Ghrelin is a growth hormone releasing acylated peptide from stomach. Nature, 402, 656-660.

51. Finn DA et al. (2005). A new look at the 5-alpha-reductase inhibitor finesteride. CNS Drug Reviews,12,1,53-76.

52. Komi PV (1992). Strength and Power in Sport. Blackwell.

53. Ricoy, J.R., A.R. Encinas, A. Cabello, S. Madero, and J. Arenas. Histochemical study of the vastus lateralis muscle fibre types of athletes. *J. Physiol. Biochem.* 54(1):41-47. 1998.

54. Staron RS et al. (2000). Fiber type composition of the vastus lateralis of young men and women. Journal of Histochemistry and Cytochemistry, 48, 623-630.

55.Suter E et al. (1993). Muscle fiber type distribution as estimated by Cybex testing and by muscle biopsy. Medicine and Science in Sport and Exercise 25,3, 363-370.

56. Douris PC et al. (2006). The relationship between maximal repetition performance and muscle fiber type as estimated by non-invasive technique of quadriceps of untrained women. Journal of Strength and Conditioning, 20,3,699-703.

57. Karp J . Designing programs that work best for your clients. Fitness Management www.fitnessmanagement.com/FM/tmpl/genPage.asp?p=/information/articles/library/features/0601features2.htmL (accessed 7/29/07).

58. Jannson E et al. (1990). Increase in the proportion of type II muscle fibers by sprint training in males. Acta Physiol Scand. 140,3,359-63.

59. Alway, S. E., P. K. et al. (1989). Regionalized adaptations and muscle fiber proliferation in stretch-induced enlargement. Journal of Applied Physiology, 66,2, 771-781.

60. Yamada, S., N. et. al. (1989). Fibroblast growth factor is stored in fiber extracellular matrix and plays a role in regulating muscle hypertrophy. Medicine and Science in Sports and Exercise. 21,5, S173-S180.

61. Schantz, P et al. (1981). The relationship between mean muscle fiber area and the muscle cross-sectional area of the thigh in subjects with large differences in thigh girth. Acta Physiol. Scand. 113: 537-539.

62. Brown LE (2007). Strength Training. National Strength & Conditioning Association. Human Kinetics.

63. Doherty T (2003). Invited interview: sarcopenia and aging. Journal of Applied Physiology, 95,1717-1727.

64. Baumgartner, RN et al. (1998). Epidemiology of sarcopenia among the elderly in New Mexico. American Journal of Epidemiology, 147,8, 755–763.

65. Greenlund, LJS et al. (2003). Sarcopenia—Consequences, mechanisms, and potential therapies. Mechanisms of Aging and Development, 124,287–299.

66. Bortz, W.M. (2001). Nonage vs. age. Journal of Gerontology: Medical Sciences 56(9): M527-M528.

67. Brooks C. Understanding sarcopenia. Fitness Management. www.fitnessmanagement.com/FM/information/articles/0906-feature3.htmL (accessed 8/18/07).

68. Sreekumaran K (2004). What is sarcopenia? Mayo Clinic. www.medicaledge.org/newspaper/n-2004october24.htmL (accessed 8/019/07).

69. Wilderson J (2004). Sarcopenia and exercise: Mechanisms, interactions and application of research findings. Strength and Conditioning Journal, 26,6, 26-31.

70. Balagopal P et al. (1997). Effects of aging on in vivo synthesis of skeletal muscle myosin heavy-chain and sarcoplasmic protein in humans. American Journal of Physiology, 273:E790–E800.

71. Schulte JN et al. (2001). Effects of resistance training on the rate of muscle protein synthesis in frail elderly people. International Journal of Sport Nutrition and Exercise Metabolism, 11:S111–S118.

72. Cannon Joe (2006). Nutritional Supplements: What Works and Why. A Review from A to Zinc –And Beyond. Available at www.Joe-Cannon.com.

73. Yarasheski KE et al. (1999). Resistance exercise training increases mixed muscle proteins synthesis in frail men and women ≥76 years old. American Journal of Physiology Endocrinology and Metabolism, 277: E118-E125.

74. Pichon C et al. (1996). Blood pressure and heart rate and metabolic cost of circuit vs. traditional weight training. Journal of Strength and Conditioning 10,3,135-156.

75. No author. What are high blood pressure and prehypertension? National Heart Lung Blood Institute. http://www.nhlbi.nih.gov/hbp/hbp/whathbp.htm (accessed 8/21/07).

76. Fleck SJ et al. (1997). Designing Resistance Training Programs, 2nd edt. Human Kinetics.

77. Fleck SJ et al. (2003). Designing Resistance Training Programs, 3rd edition. Human Kinetics.

78. Bachle TR and Earle RW (2000). Essentials of Strength Training and Conditioning, 2nd edt. Human Kinetics.

79. Drummond, MJ et al. (2005). Aerobic and resistance exercise sequence affects excess postexercise oxygen consumption. Journal of Strength and Conditioning Research, 19,2,332-337.

80. Hultman E et al. (1996). Muscle creatine loading in men. Journal of Applied Physiology 81,1,232-237.

81. Vandenberghe K et al. (1996). Caffeine counteracts the ergogenic action of muscle creatine loading. Journal of Applied Physiology, 80,452-457.

82. Hespel P (2002). Opposite actions of caffeine and creatine on muscle relaxation time in humans. Journal of Applied Physiology, 92, 512-518.

83. Mayhew D (2002). Effects of long term creatine supplementation on liver and kidney function in American college football players. International Journal of Sports Nutrition and Exercise Metabolism, 12,453-460.

84. Brosnan JT et al. (2007). Creatine: endogenous metabolite, dietary and therapeutic supplement. Annual Review of Nutrition, 27,241-261.

85. Joubert LM et al. (2006). Exercise, nutrition and homocysteine. International Journal of Sports Nutrition and Exercise Metabolism, 16,341-361.

86. McArdle, W. D., Katch, F. I., Katch, V. L. (1999). Sport & Exercise Nutrition. Lippincott, Williams & Wilkins.

87. Press release May 23 2006. Curves. New study shows curves workout can burn more than 500 calories in 30 minutes.

88. Staron RS (1991). Strength and skeletal muscle adaptations in heavy resistance trained women after detaining and retraining. Journal of Applied Physiology, 70,631-640.

89. No author. Heart attack, stroke and cardiac arrest warning signs. www.americanheart.org (accessed 9/24/07).

90. Vingren J and Krarmer WJ (2006). Effect of postexercise alcohol consumption on serum testosterone. A brief review of testosterone, resistance exercise and alcohol. Strength and Conditioning Journal, 28,1,84-87.

91. Schwab, R. et. al. (1993). Acute effects of different intensities of weight lifting on serum testosterone. Medicine and Science in Sports and Exercise, 25,12, 1381-1385.

92. Hakkien K et al. (1988). Neuromuscular and hormonal adaptations in athletes to strength training in two years. Journal of Applied Physiology, 65,2406-2412.

93. Jensen J, et al. (1991). Comparison of changes in testosterone concentrations after strength and endurance exercise in well trained men. European Journal of Applied Physiology, 63, 467-471.

94. Dressendorfer RH et al. (1991). Effects of a 15-d race on plasma steroid levels and leg muscle fitness in runners. Medicine and Science in Sports and Exercise, 23, 954-958.

95. Stone M et al. (1995). Human growth hormone: physiological functions and ergogenic efficiency, Strength and Conditioning, August, pp. 72-74.

96. Rudman D et al. (1990). Effects of human growth hormone in men over 60 years of age. New England Journal of Medicine, 323,1-6.

97. Haff GG (2006). Roundtable discussion: anabolic androgenic steroids part 1. Strength and Conditioning Journal, 28,6,42-55.

98. Kadi F (2000). Adaptations of human skeletal muscle to training and anabolic steroids. Acta Physiologica, 646 (suppl) 1-52.

99. Hickson R et al. (1990). Glucocorticoid antagonism by exercise and anabolic androgenic steroids. Medicine and Science in Sports and Exercise, 22,331-340.

100. Evans, N (2004). Current concepts in anabolic-androgenic steroids. American Journal of Sports Medicine, 32,2,534-542.

101. Parssien M et al. (2002). Steroid use and long term health risks. International Journal of Sports Medicine, 23,83-94.

102. Kraemer WJ et al .(1996). The effects of plasma cortisol evaluation on total and differential leukocyte counts in response to heavy resistance exercise. European Journal of Applied Physiology 73, 1-2, 93-97.

103. Anderson JC (2005). Stretching before and after exercise: effect on muscle soreness and injury risk. Journal of Athletic Training, 40,3 218–220.

104. Shrier, I (2005). When and whom to stretch. Gauging the Benefits and Drawbacks for Individual Patients. Physician and Sports Medicine, 33-3 www.physsportsmed.com/issues/2005/0305/shrier.htm (accessed 2/23/07).

105. Pope HG et al. (1990). Homicide and near-homicide symptoms associated with anabolic steroid use. American Journal of Psychiatry, 145, 487-490.

106. Wright KCS et al. (2002). Infant acceptance of breast milk after maternal exercise. Pediatrics 109,4, 585-589.

107. Graves JE et al. (1988). Effects of reduced training frequency on muscular strength. International Journal of Sports Medicine 9,316-319.

108. Staron, R.S., et al. (1994). Skeletal muscle adaptations during early phase of heavy-resistance training in men and women. Journal of Applied Physiology. 76,1247–1255.

109. Hakkinen, K. et al. (1988). Neuromuscular and hormonal adaptations in athletes to strength training in two years. Journal of Applied Physiology, 65, 2406–2412.

110. MacDougall, JD (1995). The time course for elevated muscle protein synthesis following heavy resistance exercise. Canadian Journal of Applied Physiology, 20,480–486.

111. Burger ME and Burger TA (2002). Neuromuscular and hormonal adaptations to resistance training: Implications for strength development in female athletes. Strength and Conditioning Journal, 24,3, 51-59.

112. Baechle TR & Earle RW (2000). Essentials of Strength and Conditioning, 2nd edt. Human Kinetics.

113. Kleiner S (2007). Power Eating, 3rd edition. Human Kinetics.

114. Foster GD et al. (2003). A randomized trial of a low carbohydrate diet for obesity. New England Journal of Medicine, 348, 2082-2090.

115. Hough, T. (1902). Ergographic studies in muscular soreness. American Journal of Physiology 7, 76-92.

116. Smith, LL (1991). Acute inflammation: the underlying mechanism in delayed onset muscle soreness? Medicine and Science in Sport and Exercise 23,5 543 - 551.

117. Friden J & Lieber RJ (1992). Structural and mechanical basis of exercise- induced muscle injury. Medicine and Science in Sport and Exercise 24,5 521-530.

118. Smith, L et al. (1993). The effects of static and ballistic stretching on delayed onset muscle soreness and creatine kinase. Research Quarterly for Exercise and Sport, 64,1, 103 - 107.

119. Sayers P (1999). The etiology of exercise induced muscle damage. Canadian Journal of Applied Physiology. 24,3,234-248.

120. Peterson J et al. (2003). Ibuprofen and acetaminophen: effect on muscle inflammation after eccentric exercise. Medicine and Science in Sports and Exercise, 35,6, 892-896.

121. Goldfarb AH (1999). Nutritional antioxidants as therapeutic and preventative modalities in exercise induced muscle damage. Canadian Journal of Applied Physiology, 24,3, 249-266.

122. Schwane JA & Armstrong RB (1983). Effects of training on skeletal muscle injury form downhill running in rats. Journal of Applied Physiology 55,3, 969- 975.

123. Myers, J et al. (2002). Exercise capacity and mortality in men referred for exercise testing. New England Journal of Medicine, 346, 11, 793-801.

124. Gulati M et al. (2005). The prognostic value of a nomogram for exercise capacity in women. New England Journal of Medicine, 353,5,468-475.

125. Gulati M et al. (2003). Exercise capacity and risk of death in women. Circulation, 108, 1554-1559. circ.ahajournals.org/cgi/content/full/108/13/1554 (accessed 12/10/07).

126. Drinkwater EJ et al. (2007). Increased number of forced repetitions does not enhance strength development with resistance training. Journal of Strength and Conditioning Research, 21,3, 841-847.

127. Barnett C et al. (1995). Effects of variations of the bench press exercise on EMG activity of five shoulder muscles. Journal of Strength and Conditioning Research, 9(4).

128. Finnie S et al. (2003). Weight lifting belt patterns among a population of health club members. Journal of Strength and Conditioning Research, 17,3,498-502.

129. Welsch E et al. (2005). Electromyographic activity of the pectoralis major and anterior deltoid muscles during three upper body lifts. Journal of Strength and Conditioning Research 19, 2, 449-452.

130. Stoutenberg M et al. (2006). Impact of foot position on electromyographical activity of the superficial quadriceps muscle during leg extension. Journal of Strength and Conditioning Research, 19,4, 931-938.

131. Chandler JT and Stone MH (1991). The squat exercise in athletic conditioning: A position statement and review of the literature. Strength and Conditioning Journal, 13,51-60.

132. Gardner PJ and Cole D (1999). The Stiff Leg Dead Lift. Strength and Conditioning Journal, 21,5,7-14

133. Safran M et al. Instructions for Sports Medicine Patients. Elsevier Publishers.

134. Ross MD (2002). Addressing calf muscle weakness following anterior cruciate ligament reconstruction. Strength and Conditioning Journal, 24,1, 71-72.

135. Antonio J (2000). Nonuniform response of skeletal muscle to heavy resistance training: can bodybuilders induce regional muscle hypertrophy? Journal of Strength and Conditioning Research, 14,1 102-113.

136. Green C M et al. (2007). Effect of grip width on bench press on bench press performance and risk of injury. Strength and Conditioning Journal, 29,5,10-14.

137. Berger A (1991).Effect of tonic neck reflex in the bench press. Journal of Applied Sports Science Research, 5,4,188-191.

138. Levy AM and Fuerst ML (1993). Sports Injury Handbook: Professional Advice for Amateur Athletes. Wiley.

139. Sternlicht E et al. (2007). Electromyographic comparison of stability ball crunch with a traditional crunch. Journal of Strength and Conditioning Research, 21,2,506-509.

140. Crate T (June 1997). Analysis of the lat pull down. Strength and Conditioning, 76.

141. ACSM (1997). ACSM's Exercise Management for Persons with Chronic Diseases and Disabilities. Human Kinetics.

142. Gettman LR et a (1981). Circuit weight training: a critical review of its physiological benefits. The physician and Sports Medicine, 9,44-60

143. Gotshalk, LA et al. (2004). Cardiovascular responses to a high-volume continuous circuit resistance training protocol. Journal of Strength and Conditioning Research, 18,4 760-764.

144. Humburg H et al. (2007). 1 set vs. 3 set resistance training: a crossover study. Journal of Strength and Conditioning Research, 21,2 578-582.

145. Hass CJ et al. (2000). Single vs. multiple sets in long term recreational weightlifters. Medicine and Science in Sports and Exercise, 32,235-242.

146. Calder AW et al. (1994). Comparison of whole and split weight raining routines in young women. Canadian Journal of Applies Physiology, 19,2,185-199.

147. Higbie EJ et al. (1996). Effect of concentric and eccentric training on muscle strength cross sectional area and neural activation. Journal of Applied Physiology, 812173-2181.

148. Keogh J et al. (1999). A cross sectional comparison of different resistance training techniques in the bench press. Journal of Strength and Conditioning Research, 13,3,247-258.

149. Hunter GR et al. (2003). Comparison of metabolic and heart rate responses to super slow vs. traditional resistance training. Journal of Strength and Conditioning Specialists, 17,1,76-81.

150. Keeler LK et al. (2001). Early phase adaptations of training speed vs. superslow resistance training on strength and aerobic capacity in sedentary individuals. Journal of Strength and Conditioning Research, 15, 309-314.

151. Doan BK et al. (2002). Effects of increased eccentric loading on bench press 1RM. Journal of Strength and Conditioning Research, 16,1, 9-13.

152. Brudvig TJ (2007). Identification of the signs and symptoms of acute exertional rhabdomyolysis in athletes: a guide for the practitioner. Strength and Conditioning Journal, 29,1,10-14.

153. Springer BL et al. (2003). Two cases of exertional rhabdomyolysis precipitated by personal trainers. Medicine and Science in sports and exercise,35, 9,1499-1502.

154. Brown B (2004). Exertional Rhabdomyolysis. Physician and Sports Medicine, 34,4.

155. Kao PF et al. (2004). Rectus abdominis rhabdomyolysis after sit ups: unexpected detection by bone scan. British Journal of Sports Medicine, 32,3,253-254.

156. American Heart Association. www.americanheart.org.

157. Wansink B (2006). Mindless Eating.

158. Joubert LM et al. (2006). Exercise, nutrition and homocysteine. International Journal of Sports Medicine and Exercise Metabolism, 16,341-361.

159. Robergs RA & Landwehr R (May 2002). The surprising history of the "HRmax = 220-age" equation. Journal of Exercise Physiology Online, Vol 5, No 2.

160. Bariatric Surgery. In. University of Southern California. Center for colorectal and pelvic floor disorders. www.surgery.usc.edu/divisions/cr/bariatricsurgery.htmL (accessed 4/8/08).

161. Discovery Health CME: Bariatric Surgery. Weighing the Options. April 7 2007 www.discoveryhealthcme.discovery.com.

162. National Heart, Lung, and Blood Institute, National Institutes of Health (2000). The Practical Guide: Identification, Evaluation, and Treatment of Overweight and Obesity in Adults (NIH Publication No. 00-4084). www.nhlbi.nih.gov/guidelines/obesity/prctgd_c.pdf (accessed 4/7/08).

163. McLean KP et al. (1992). Validity of Futrex-5000 for Body Composition. Medicine and Exercise in Sports and Exercise, 2,.2, 253-257.

164. Seventh report of the Joint National Committee on Prevention, Detection, Evaluation and Treatment of High Blood Pressure. US department of health and human services. www.nhlbi.nih.gov/guidelines/hypertension/jnc7full.htm (accessed 4/17/08).

165. Payne G et al. (1993). Exercise and Vo2max in children: A meta-analysis. Research Quarterly for Exercise and Sport, 64,305-313.

166. Falk B et al. (1996). The effects of resistance and martial arts training in 6-8 year old boys. Pediatric Exercise Science, 8,48-56.

167. Kelly AKW (2005). Practical exercise advice during pregnancy. Physician and Sports Medicine, 33,6. www.physsportsmed.com/issues/2005/0605/weiss.htm (accessed 3/5/08).

168. Sternfeld B et al. (1995). Exercise during pregnancy and pregnancy outcome. Medicine and Science in Sports and Exercise, 27,5,634-640.

169. Clapp JF et al. (1990). Neonatal morphometrics after endurance exercise during pregnancy. American Journal of Obstetrics and Gynecology, 163(6 pt 1):1805-1811.

170. Depken D (1996). Exercise during pregnancy. Concerns for fitness professionals. Strength and Conditioning Journal. October. pp. 43-51.

171. Ireland ML et al. (2000). The effects of pregnancy on the musculoskeletal system. Clinical Orthopedics and Related Research, 372(Mar):169-179.

172. Gerben C (2007). Deep venous thrombosis, upper extremity. E Medicine. ww.emedicine.com/radio/topic774.htm (accessed 3/15/08).

173. Pujol TJ et al. (2007). Resistance training during pregnancy. Strength and Conditioning Journal 29,2, 44-46.

174. Wolf L (1993). In: Skinner JS. Exercise Testing and Exercise Prescription for Special Cases. Lea & Febiger.

175. Gau G. VLDL: What is it? www.mayclinic.com (accessed 5/4/08).

176. Ronai P (2008). Resistance training for persons with osteoarthritis and rheumatoid arthritis. Journal of Strength and Conditioning, 30, 2, 32-34.

177. Ehlke K (2006). Resistance exercise for post myocardial infarction patients: current guidelines and future considerations, Journal of Strength and Conditioning, 28,6, 56-62.

178. Waller, M (2000). Strength and conditioning in multiple sclerosis patients. Strength and Conditioning Journal, 22,2,40-41.

179. No authors. What Causes MS? National Multiple Sclerosis. www.nationalmssociety.org (accessed 5/12/08).

180. No authors. Prednisone. Medline Plus. www.nlm.nih.gov/medlineplus/druginfo/medmaster/a601102.htmL (accessed 5/12/08).

181. Willardson JM (2008). A brief review: how much rest between sets? Journal of Strength and Conditioning, 30,3, 44-50.

182. Phillips SM et al. (2007). A critical examination of dietary protein requirements, benefits and excess in athletes. International Journal of Sports Nutrition and Exercise Metabolism, 17,S58-S76.

183. Stone M et al. (2006). Stretching: acute and chronic. The potential consequences. Journal of Strength and Conditioning Research, 28,6, 66-74.

184. No authors. Exertional Rhabdomyolysis and Acute Renal Impairment -New York City and Massachusetts, 1988. Morbidity and Mortality Weekly Report. October 26, 1990, 39,42,751-756.

185. Friery, K (2008). Incidence of disease and injury in former athletes: a review. Journal of Exercise Physiology, Online, 11,2, 26-45.

186. Kravitz, L (2005) Lactate: Not Guilty As Charged. IDEA Fitness Journal, 2 (3) 23-25.

187. Wen et.al. (2011). Minimum amount of physical activity for reduced mortality and extended life expectancy: A prospective cohort study. Lancet,378 (9798), 1244-1253.

188. ACSM's Guidliens for Exercise Testing and Prescription, 7th edt.

189.Cole, C et al (1999). Heart-Rate Recovery Immediately after Exercise as a Predictor of Mortality. New England Journal of Medicine, 341:1351-1357.

189. ACSM's Guidliens for Exercise Testing and Prescription, 8th edt.

190. Cadore, EL, et. al (2012). Hormonal responses to concurrent strength and endurance training with different exercise orders. Journal of Strenght and Conditioning Research, 26,12, 3281-3288.

191. Flan, KL et al (2011). Muscle damage and muscle remodeling: no pain, no gain? Journal of Experimental Biology, 214 (pt4),674-679.

192. Schoenfeld, B (2011). Does cardio after an overnight fast maximize fat loss? Journal of Strength and Conditioning, 33,1,:23-25

193. Yamaguci et al (2005). Effects of static stretching for 30 seconds and dynamic stretching on leg extension power. Journal of Strength and Conditioning Research, 9,3,677-683.

194. WebMd.com. Testosterone. Accessed 8/19/14.

Index

and energy metabolism, 23
    and muscle fatigue, 23
lateral, defined, 28
leptin, defined, 30
ligaments, 31

M

macrocycle, defined, 85
macronutrients, 20
manager on duty (MOD), 177
marketing, 181
maximum heart rate, estimating, 144
medial, defined, 27
mesomorph, 164
metabolic equivalents, 150
metabolic syndrome, 193
METs, 150
MI, defined, 191
mitochondria, exercise adaptations, 21
mitral valve, 61
motor unit, defined, 43
multiple sclerosis, exercise guidelines, 198
muscle confusion, 181
muscle fiber types, 45
    gender differences, 48
    percentage of, 47
muscle mass, estimating, 170
muscle memory, 53
muscle spindle, defined, 31
muscle tissue, types, 29
muscular endurance
    and push-up test, 156
    defined, 156
    training guidelines, 82
myofibrils, 40
myoglobin, defined, 45
myosin, defined, 40
myostatin and muscle growth, 50

N

near infrared interactance, 169
negatives, defined, 53
nervous system
    central vs. peripheral, 66
    sympathetic vs. parasympathetic, 66
neuromuscular junction, 43
neuropathy, 194
nitric oxide supplements, 64

O

obesity
    and BMI, 163
    and metabolism, 183
    and morbid orbesity, 163
    defined, 163
OBLA, 24
older adult, exercise guidelines, 203
organs, defined, 29
osteoarthritis, defined, 30

osteoblast cells, 35
osteopenia, 197
osteoporosis, exercise guidelines, 197
overload principle, 73
overtraining syndrome, 171
oxygen debt, 26

P

PAR-Q, 9
percent maximum heart rate formula, when not to use, 148
percent of maximum heart rate formula, 144
periodization, periods and phases of, 85
peripheral artery disease (PAD), 182
personal training
    and sexual harassment, 182
    and touching clients, 13
    average annual salary, 2
    degree vs. certification, 3
    dress code, 1
    email address, 6
    fitness director, 177
    health club compensation models, 15
    innapropriate behavior, 2
    interviewing skills, 182
    liability insurance, 10
    making a good impression with clients, 12
    precautions for female trainers, 182
    resume, 182
    self-employed compensation models, 16
    tracking finances, 18
plantar fasciitis, 126
plantarflexion, defined, 28
posterior, defined, 28
pregnancy, exercise guidelines, 205
prehypertension, defined, 65
preload, defined, 67
pronation, defined, 28
protein, use during exercise, 25
pulse, measuring, 64
push-up test, 156

R

rate pressure product, 65
red blood cells and cigarettes, 59
repetition maximum, 153
    10 RM test, 153
residual volume, defined, 61
respiratory exchange ratio (RER), 71
resting heart rate
    and exercise, 66
    and health risk, 171
    and overtraining syndrome, 171
    average, 171
    how to take, 171e
Rhabdomyolysis, 57
RICE, defined, 183
RM, defined, 79
Rockport walking test, 160
rotator cuff, 106
    and impingement syndrome, 107

About Joe Cannon

Joe Cannon, MS, is an exercise physiologist, personal trainer, and health educator. He holds an MS degree in Exercise Science and a BS degree in Chemistry & Biology. He is doubly certified by the National Strength & Conditioning Association (NSCA) as a Certified Strength and Conditioning Specialist (CSCS) and as a Personal Trainer (NSCA-CPT).

A dynamic and motivational speaker who specializes in presenting information in easy-to-understand terms, Joe has been educating fitness trainers since 1995. As the Director of Wellness for a health club that ranked among the top 100 of all clubs in the United States, he designed and implemented groundbreaking exercise programs for a diverse range of individuals including seniors as well as those with cancer, osteoporosis, fibromyalgia, and developmental disabilities.

For more information about personal training, fitness, and health, or to contact Joe directly, go to his website:

www.Joe-Cannon.com

Other Books by Joe Cannon

1. ***Nutrition Essentials***: An information-packed nutrition and sports nutrition textbook that was designed specifically to address the needs and questions of fitness professionals and to help them study and prepare for *any* sports nutrition certification. *Nutrition Essentials* is the companion text to Joe cannon's book on Personal Fitness Training.

2. ***Nutritional Supplements: What Works and Why***: A no-nonsense, A to Z review of 119 vitamins, minerals, herbs, and other supplements. This book cuts through the hype and deciphers what works and what does not work, basing all conclusions on scientific facts and rational thought. Over 400 pages in length, this book also highlights side effects of which few people in the world are aware. An eye-opening must-read for everyone in the fitness industry! Easy-to-read and highly referenced, this book is the culmination of over 15 years of Joe Cannon's study and investigation of dietary supplements.

3. ***Personal Fitness Training: Beyond the Basics***: The perfect book to help people study and prepare for *any* personal training certification. Joe Cannon reviews not only the essential exercise science topics of personal fitness training, but also how to apply that knowledge in the real world. This book also covers real-life issues that fitness professionals encounter each day. Essentially, this is a college-level textbook that cuts out the technical jargon that most trainers do not need while focusing on what they should know. The emphasis of the book is to provide people with the knowledge needed to work effectively and safely with people and to help trainers outshine their competition.

4. ***Personal Trainer's Big Book of Questions and Answers***: This book provides accurate answers to over 135 of the most popular exercise, nutrition, and general health questions that fitness professionals are asked every day. This book was created from actual questions that fitness trainers and lay persons have asked Joe Cannon over the years. This is an e-book that can be easily downloaded from Joe Cannon's website.

For more information, or to order any of these books, visit www.Joe-Cannon.com.

Made in the USA
San Bernardino, CA
28 April 2020